REVOLUTIONARY GRANDPARENTS

REVOLUTIONARY GRANDPARENTS

Generations Healing Autism with Love and Hope

**COLLECTED BY HELEN CONROY
AND LISA JOYCE GOES**

Foreword by Dan Burton

Skyhorse Publishing

Skyhorse Publishing books may be purchased in bulk at special discounts for sales promotion, corporate gifts, fund-raising, or educational purposes. Special editions can also be created to specifications. For details, contact the Special Sales Department, Skyhorse Publishing, 307 West 36th Street, 11th Floor, New York, NY 10018 or info@skyhorsepublishing.com.

Skyhorse® and Skyhorse Publishing® are registered trademarks of Skyhorse Publishing, Inc.®, a Delaware corporation.

Visit our website at www.skyhorsepublishing.com.

10 9 8 7 6 5 4 3 2 1

Library of Congress Cataloging-in-Publication Data is available on file.

Cover design by Rain Saukas
Cover photos: iStockphoto

Print ISBN: 978-1-5107-0538-8
Ebook ISBN: 978-1-5107-0540-1

Printed in the United States of America

Dedicated to all Grandparents who have walked beside us on our journey, supporting and loving their children and grandchildren through the ups and downs of autism.

Contents

Foreword

ONE OF THE BIGGEST TRAGEDIES THE HUMAN RACE HAS HAD TO FACE in recent history is the epidemic of autism. Much of the heartache that many parents and grandparents have had to face could have been eliminated if our health agencies had done a better job.

When I was Chairman of the Government Reform and Oversight Committee in the US House of Representatives, I had many hearings on autism. There was very strong evidence that mercury in children's vaccines was one of the causes of autism. For whatever reason, the health agencies in America closed their eyes to the evidence that was uncovered in those hearings.

I am convinced that thimerosal, the mercury preservative in children's vaccines, is a contributing factor in this epidemic. In my opinion, all parents should try to find vaccines in single shot vials that are thimerosal-free. Four years of hearings on this issue, which included testimonials from doctors and scientists from around the world, should not be ignored.

I want to thank the authors of this book for working so hard to bring this issue to the attention of parents and grandparents everywhere.

Congressman Dan Burton, Retired

Introduction

WHEN MY SON HARRY AND I LEFT THE DEVELOPMENTAL PEDIATRI-
cian's office with an autism and probable apraxia diagnosis in hand
almost six years ago, I had a heavy, heavy heart. It wasn't because I
understood the full implications of autism or how it would change
us as a family, since I did not. It wasn't because I realized I would
come to spend on treatments many times over what we had spent
purchasing a home. It also wasn't because I mourned the friends he
might never have, the college he might never attend, the jobs he
might never hold. No, none of those things. My heart was heavy
because the doctor left me without hope.

"Do the best you can, for as long as you can, and then . . ." Then,
he implied, we would need to look into institutionalizing my son,
my sweet, beautiful angel. I questioned the doctor about things I had
read but was told that diets didn't work and intensive biomedical
interventions could be deadly. I was told to just survive, to do my
duty for as long as I could. The doctor also told me that I shouldn't
feel guilty when the time inevitably came to turn my son over to a
stranger's care.

As I drove away from the office, I looked at my son in the rear-
view mirror. I was so sad. But I was mourning a loss that hadn't
occurred. Harry was still very much alive. He was, my mother

reminded me, the same child I had brought into the office a few hours earlier, hoping that this physician could tell me what was wrong and how to fix it. The same child I loved with all my heart. The same child I had held, and rocked, and whispered sweet words to the night before. So instead of handing my hope over to a white-coated grim reaper, I vowed to cling to it with every shred of my strength.

I looked back at his beautiful face, smiling at the movie playing on the car's DVD player, and I made a promise to never give up on him.

No one in my family had any experience with autism. It became my job to relentlessly research the disease and become the expert to guide my family in what to do. My even more important job, however, was to hold hope high, to share it with everyone, to let them know that we would find our way together. It became my job to hold the lantern in the dark and guide us all along the unlit passageways, reassuring everyone we would eventually find the way out.

When I talk to families with a newly diagnosed child, the first thing I always say is "There is so much hope." Because there is. Hope is the one thing you absolutely have to have on this journey. Money and a bit of luck are great, but without hope your path will be much more difficult.

The other critical pillar is family support. Harry's four grandparents have all played pivotal roles in his development. We are very blessed that they all believed in what we were doing and took on parts of his care. All of them have a special relationship with him; all of them have paid for treatments; all of them have watched him when we needed a break. They have cooked for him, tickled and wrestled him, done therapy with him, and considered him as capable as his siblings. We know how lucky we are, and we are so grateful that they are so committed to his life and well-being.

In this book, you will hear from a number of grandparents who are similarly committed to their grandchildren with autism. These families amaze me, and I am humbled by their stories of love and compassion.

Our hope for grandparents new to the autism diagnosis is that they will read this book with an open heart and follow the words of wisdom from their peers who have walked this path before them. I often think that, in some ways, a grandparent has a harder time dealing with this diagnosis than the parent.

No grandparent should have to grieve silently as they watch their child's life fall apart while they mourn the loss of a grandchild. One in seventeen grandparents is now affected by autism. Chances are, many of your golf buddies and bridge partners are among those affected. Start talking about autism in your community. Dig in with your son or daughter. Become involved and committed. We promise to be there to support you as you have supported us.

With much love,
The Thinking Moms' Revolution

Helen Conroy

1

Bubby
The Power of Play

THERE ARE MOMENTS IN LIFE WHEN TIME STOPS AND YOU KNOW THAT your world has changed so completely that nothing will ever be the same again. I experienced one of these moments when my daughter phoned and told me between tears that she was sure that our seven-month-old grandson Ri was autistic. At first I challenged her and refused to believe the behavior—or rather, lack of behavior—she described meant that Ri was autistic. He was our miracle baby. How could he be autistic?

Our daughter had several miscarriages before the doctors finally discovered she had a blood disorder related to vitamin B12 and an inability to convert B12 into the methylated form that can be used by the body. This disorder caused blood clots to form during pregnancy. Eventually a solution was found. Although it was a high-risk pregnancy for both mother and child, our miracle baby was born. We were ecstatic. He was a beautiful baby. My husband and I stayed for two weeks after Ri was born to help out; then we drove back to our home eight hours away. We were long-distance grandparents. It was very difficult to leave our grandson, but we were determined to form a lasting relationship with him and visit as often as possible. I did not know then that it would be several years before Ri recognized me as his Bubby. (That's the Yiddish word for grandmother.)

There were some early signs that something was amiss. Ri had absolutely no interest in people. He avoided eye contact at all costs—he would move his head just to avoid meeting someone's eyes. He screamed if his hands or feet were touched. In general, it seemed like he was asleep with his eyes open.

When Ri was twelve months old, the pediatrician agreed to have him tested at my daughter's insistence. Two people from Early Intervention Services came to observe Ri playing at home. Our daughter said that Ri was quite enamored with the younger of the two women and, for the first time in months, was focused and played normally. He laughed, made a little eye contact, and even sat in the woman's lap. The observers felt that he was a normal healthy baby and told our daughter not to worry. When they left, however, he returned to his regular, placid, and unreachable demeanor.

The periods when he was absent, just staring into space, became longer and longer. He was easily upset and had meltdowns for no apparent reason. It became difficult to take him grocery shopping or to the mall because of his meltdowns. Even going from upstairs to downstairs prompted a daily thirty-minute meltdown. My daughter continued to take Ri to the storytelling time at the library, play dates, the park, and children's birthday parties, but she could see that his development was falling further and further behind the development of neurotypical children. She called me daily, her voice filled with concern. All I could do was listen, since we were long-distance grandparents. I could not drop by and give her a break so she could take a bath, go to the gym, or go for a walk to clear her head.

When Ri was fourteen months old, the family came to visit us in Canada for a week. On the second day of the visit, Ri started to cry and would not stop for what seemed like hours. His dad took him upstairs to calm him down, and Ri continued to cry until he fell asleep, exhausted. His dad felt that Ri wanted to go home, and when he realized he was not going home immediately, he had a meltdown. It was a very difficult day for all of us, because we could see that something was terribly wrong. Ri was not improving; he was getting worse.

When he was eighteen months old, my daughter and son-in-law took Ri to a specialized clinic to be tested again. This time the results were devastating! The doctors predicted that Ri would never recognize his parents, never be able to function on his own, and never even be able to follow simple directions. They said he would probably need to be institutionalized when he was older and that there were "some very nice institutions nowadays." They gave my daughter and son-in-law a pamphlet from Autism Speaks and sent them home completely traumatized.

How could this be? What could be done? How could we, Ri's grandparents, help change this terrible diagnosis and make everything better? We thought we couldn't; we thought no one could. Fortunately, our daughter is a fighter! She started researching what services were available in her community and signed Ri up for Early Intervention Services. For Ri, these services included ABA (applied behavior analysis) and occupational therapy. Our daughter worked with Ri as well to support the work of the professionals. They did repetitive exercises, such as pointing to the correct object, putting together a four-piece puzzle, jumping on a trampoline, and trying to catch a rolling ball. Quite often, Ri was frustrated and had meltdowns, not understanding what was expected of him. He was confused. He did not recognize us or his parents. He did not respond to his name. He repeated episodes from children's TV shows over and over, not understanding what he was saying at all.

And yet, despite all of this, Ri had a wonderful personality. He enjoyed dancing to music, playing his drums, and—when he was not having a meltdown or hiding in his own world—he had a mischievous smile. He loved his *My Baby Can Read* videos and could read at eighteen months, though he did not understand what he read. He also loved Thomas the Train shows and toy trains. But Ri did not play with his trains like other children his age. He banged them together or lined them up over and over again. Ri also spent hours counting from one to twenty both forwards and backwards. He must be bright, we thought; otherwise, how could he read and count? It was all very confusing.

When we visited, we had to tiptoe around the house for two to three hours before he would acknowledge that we were in the house and accept our presence. Sometimes, inadvertently, I said or did something that irritated Ri, and he responded by crying and screaming for five to ten minutes before we could calm him down. Once, he took my hand and started leading me somewhere. I was excited, thinking he wanted to play with me. Sadly, he led me to the front door. He wanted me to leave his house, because he had no idea who I was or that I had come to play with him. During another visit, Ri took his Zaidy's (grandfather's) hand and walked him to the front door. My husband was crushed.

Our daughter and son-in-law saw that ABA was not working for Ri. It was only making him angry and causing him to withdraw even more into his own world. Our daughter continued her search for a therapy with a different approach. One day she phoned us, quite excited. She had found a behavioral program called the Son-Rise Program[1] that was specifically developed for children with autism. What was so amazing about this call is that on that same day I had been looking for similar programs in Canada. I had heard of the Reena Foundation in Canada for developmental problems, and my Google search for Reena kept

---

1   The Son-Rise Program is a play therapy method in which the parent (or grandparent) runs the program from their home. For more information, visit http://www.autismtreatmentcenter.org.

showing the Son-Rise Program in the US. I went to their site and was just starting to read about it when my daughter telephoned. Talk about coincidence! This had to be a good sign.

My daughter was sure the Son-Rise Program would help. What she liked about its approach was that you, the parent, play with the child and "join" in their repetitive play. Instead of prohibiting their repetitive behaviors, you use them to show your child that you are interested in their world and share their interests. Eventually, your child notices that you enjoy and want to participate in their activities. After you join your child in their world, you slowly begin to offer them the opportunity to get involved in yours, using whatever motivates them, no matter what it is. This, of course, takes years, but Son-Rise had videos that showed how over time the program could improve the quality of life for the whole family. Our daughter convinced us that this approach could work. Best of all, we, the long-distance grandparents, could help by being volunteers on Ri's Son-Rise Program team.

My daughter went to Massachusetts for the five-day Son-Rise Program Start-Up to learn how to set up a playroom, gather volunteers, lead team meetings, set manageable goals, and play with her son in a way that would inspire growth. She explained to us what needed to be done. By that point, my husband and I were both retired, so we came and helped set up the playroom by moving furniture, setting up high shelves, and buying some of the equipment. Soon the room was ready. I was the first volunteer. I watched Ri and my daughter play together via a webcam that was set up in the playroom and learned how to handle his meltdowns, follow his lead, and play the way he played, even if it was not how kids usually played. There was so much to learn, but I did it! Our daughter hired several wonderful college students (with no experience with autism) and trained them in Son-Rise as well.

Ri loved the alphabet, counting, and naming the American states and their capitals. So, as a volunteer, I learned to love those things too. Ri and his team spent weeks counting and repeating the alphabet because that was what Ri liked to do. Gradually, he began to look into my eyes more often when he wanted another toy or when he wanted me to say the next number. After hours of play, he started to play a game a bit differently or use a toy in a new way. For example, the Son-Rise Team spent six hours a day for two weeks just watching Ri put together an ABC puzzle. They weren't allowed to speak or participate to make sure Ri didn't have a meltdown. So they silently cheered him on by raising their hands in the air to show they supported his repetitive behavior. Gradually they were allowed to quietly cheer him on. Then one day our daughter tried to hand him a puzzle piece. When she had tried to do this in the past, he screamed, cried, and grabbed the piece; this time he looked at her briefly and smiled. Over the next month the team built up the activity to where they were taking turns with Ri putting the puzzle together. We were making progress, and because I came to visit for a week every six weeks, I could really see the improvements. He enjoyed the play-room and actually dragged me in to play with him, not out the door to leave his house. The Son-Rise Program was working!

Now when we came to visit, we no longer needed to tiptoe around the house for hours. One day, about a year into the pro-gram, my grandson spontaneously turned to me and said, "I love you, Bubby!" The tears welled up in my eyes. Ri knew who I was and wanted to be with me! Ri now also recognized his parents and my husband, and he felt secure with us and his Son-Rise Team. Another miracle!

In Ri's case, there is one more piece to the puzzle of his autism. At around the same time Ri first told me he loved me, my daughter took him to a DAN! (Defeat Autism Now!) doctor. A series of blood tests showed that Ri's methylation cycle was all messed up, which meant that his body could not metabolize vitamin B12 into its meth-ylated state, MB12. This vitamin is crucial for the development of brain cells and the functioning of the brain and nervous system, so

Ri now receives daily injections, given by his parents, of methylated B12. The DAN! doctor stated that some kind of therapy program and methylated B12 injections are both required to help Ri recover from autism. The Son-Rise Program started his recovery, and the methyl B12 shots significantly sped up the process!

Meanwhile, magic was happening in the playroom. The team enthusiastically participated as Ri scripted his own TV shows. We waited for moments of opportunity (when we felt a connection) to ask a question or change the story slightly; over time, Ri started to answer those questions and made more room for our suggestions. These interactions grew and grew until the team was creating entirely new stories together. We used specially tailored games and our energy and enthusiasm to teach him how to do all kinds of things, like making and reading facial expressions and creating new stories of his own. We never pushed him to perform; instead, we waited until he was ready to engage. The only reward was the human interaction itself, and we eventually taught Ri how to be a friend by modeling friendship for him.

Approximately two and a half years after starting the Son-Rise Program, Ri had completed all of its stages. He is an inquisitive, happy child. He knows how to calm himself down when having a meltdown (though he rarely has these anymore), and he plays with a wide variety of toys properly instead of just banging them together. He talks in sentences and responds to questions and to his name. We have conversations together, and he is interested in us. He enjoys baking cakes, playing soccer, and doing science experiments with his mommy. He goes to a regular pre-school, has friends, and arranges play dates. He even asked to have a Halloween party at his house this year and insisted on inviting the whole class.

Who needs scientific proof that Son-Rise works when these words say it all: "I love you, mommy and daddy," "I love you, Bubby and Zaidy." I can even talk to him on the phone! Granted, there are still some mountains to climb. Though he is fully verbal, Ri has to undergo speech therapy to help strengthen the muscles in his mouth, and his Daddy practices his exercises with him every night with tremendous results. Ri also receives occupational therapy to overcome weakness in his other muscles. He is making progress here also. Sometimes he has a little trouble focusing and can seem a bit scattered, but he loves to play and chat, share his feelings, and ask questions. He is a really charming little boy.

During the last visit to see the DAN! doctor, my daughter was told that Ri did not exhibit any signs of autism! His ATEC[2] score, which started out at 154, is now 2. (The higher the number, the more significant the autism. Anything below 10 is considered neurotypical.) We are so lucky to have found the right combination of biomedical and behavioral programs for our miracle grandchild!

Thank goodness for the Son-Rise Program, Ri's Son-Rise Team members, DAN! doctors, our loyal, loving son-in-law, and our courageous, persistent, hopeful, brilliant daughter. It was daunting going into Ri's program for the first time, but I am so glad that I got to witness and be a part his journey out of autism.

Final update:

Today, at six and a half, Ri is in a regular first-grade class at a private school. He is continuing to develop and mature. He enjoys reading, building Lego sets, writing stories and comics, learning robotics, and just having fun! He also has arranged a few play dates with his classmates at school. His passion for life, cheerful disposition, inquisitive nature and playfulness continue to amaze me.

Bubby
(Friend of Team TMR)

---

2   The Autism Treatment Evaluation Checklist is a tool for tracking the progress of autistic individuals. It can be found online at http://www. autism.com/ind_atec.

2

Pop

Finding the Proverbial Happy Ending

MY OLDEST CHILD WAS BORN IN ARLINGTON, TEXAS, ON FEBRUARY 5, 1967. I took my wife Marsha to the hospital around one or two in the morning, excited and a little nervous, but not terribly anxious because I had seen my mother go through this several times, and she always treated it like a trip to the grocery store. I'm the oldest of my mother's seven children. All of my siblings were delivered fat and happy. What could go wrong?

So when my daughter Kim announced she was pregnant with our first grandchild, there was no fear or anxiety, only joy and anticipation. On the night Kim went into labor with Patrick, I was in Greenville, South Carolina, at a Michelin tire dealer meeting. I was an independent tire dealer for decades. Marsha had cautioned me about going to the meeting when Kim was due to give birth, but the first one is usually late, so I went anyway. Kim was in Atlanta only a few hours away, so if it happened, I could get there quickly.

Well, I got the call at about 2:00 a.m. on Sunday morning and made it to Atlanta before daylight. Patrick was born on September 24, 2000, and except for his mother's damaged tail bone, the delivery was unremarkable. My mood was marked by a sense of gratitude that my daughter had grown up smart and beautiful, married a man who loved her, and delivered to her parents this extraordinary grandchild. This was another chapter in a story that could not conceivably avoid the proverbial happy ending.

Sam and Kim had both graduated from the University of Georgia. Both had successfully worked in their degree fields in Atlanta. If a parent had written a script for their child to follow, this is how the script would have read. As the oldest of seven, I had a childhood that was more about survival than nurture. But my grandchild's life would be guided by mature, well-educated parents, who were well read in the art and science of parenting.

After Patrick was born, I still had employees who lived and worked in Atlanta, so I spent the day there at least twice a month. I remember the first time I brought Patrick home with me. Marsha and I lived in Statesboro, about three hours away. Patrick was about six months old, sitting in the back seat, seeming to enjoy the ride, and unconcerned that I had taken him away from his mother and father. He appeared to be comfortable with Marsha and me, but it was surprising that he did not notice the absence of his parents.

I can't say that Marsha and I noticed anything peculiar about Patrick in the early months, but I remember at some point telling a friend that Patrick was not interested in engaging with others. At the time, I didn't think his uninterruptable behavior was obsessive, but in retrospect I'm sure it was. Exactly when he began to display symptoms, I'm not sure. I remember vaguely telling his mother that he must have a hearing problem, and that she should have his hearing checked. When his name was called, he was completely unresponsive. Ultimately, she did take him to the doctor, and we were devastated by the news. Patrick, the focus of our lives for the first three years of his life, had AUTISM.

But they called it PDD-NOS (pervasive developmental disorder-not otherwise specified), not autism. I guess they tell everybody that. Break it to them gently. Looking back, I realize that the signs of autism were unavoidable to the trained eye. We were untrained. Now, seeing other children walk on tiptoes, avoid eye contact, lose their speech, and not respond to parents and others causes a big, helpless, empty feeling.

Several months ago, I saw a parent on TV attempting to "show off" his young son. The child appeared to be violently avoiding eye contact, and not necessarily to see something outside the view of the camera. He became unruly just to avoid eye contact. I hope I was wrong about the child's apparent symptoms, but I still had that big, helpless, empty feeling.

As a parent or grandparent who knows the telltale signs, you frequently see children with behaviors that could be symptomatic. Walking on tiptoes and lack of eye contact are not definite symptoms, and I've seen children who did not have age-appropriate speech but were completely neurotypical. Knowledge of symptoms frequently leads to internal conflicts.

Should I tell the parents? If I'm wrong, they will never forgive me. If I'm correct, I will send their lives into an interminable tailspin, making them feel like an airplane that is spinning out of control, but never hits the ground.

You never crash. You exist in this constant dizzying spin that keeps your life in an unrelenting state of unease. Things around you are never settled enough to allow a fixed point of reference. Unless you are one of the lucky ones whose child loses their diagnosis, it's a life sentence.

My neighbor has a degree in early childhood education. I'm certain she knew Patrick had autism or some severe developmental disorder long before his diagnosis. She chose not to reveal what she knew. I could not imagine why at the time. Now, I understand. I have sympathy for the conflict she must have experienced. There is no blood test or x-ray that can confirm diagnosis. Whether your child is high functioning or severe and nonverbal, a diagnosis is decided by grading various observed behaviors. And when and if you are given a diagnosis, because the evaluation of behaviors is so subjective and the symptoms so varied, few parents will say, "Now I know what I'm dealing with." They surely never say, "Now I know how to start the healing."

No one leaves the doctor's office with the following words: "Mr. and Mrs. Jones, your son has autism. He's somewhere around point 'A' on the spectrum. Children around point 'A' generally do best with protocol 'A' described in this pamphlet. This protocol includes the following diet, exercise, and therapies. Here are the ones I think your insurance will pay for." None of that happens. It's not like cancer or a car wreck.

In the case of cancer, if it's a more treatable form, after the anger and denial pass, you begin to think, "I can beat this." You think, "I have a course of treatment, my chances of remission are high." Not the case with autism. Rarely will you hear a best-case scenario. You can look forward to decades of never-ending therapies. And if you ask, "Will he ever marry, go to college, live independently, have a normal life?" you are likely to get a weak "Well, it's possible." Israel is more optimistic about peace in the Middle East.

One of the most frustrating things about autism is that symptoms are so varied in nature and severity. And the various therapies are even more numerous. Kim has often told me stories about therapies that have had remarkable results for a child or children, only to be disheartened to find that the benefits are not universal. In fact, I don't know of any therapy that is universally successful, except the gluten-free/casein-free diet. It's relatively easy to follow, and I think most would see immediate benefit. For the most part, however, matching therapies to your child for best effect is frustrating and at times must seem impossible.

The tenacity required is physically, mentally, emotionally, and financially bankrupting.

Before Patrick's father Sam became as successful as he is now, Marsha and I helped significantly with the cost of Patrick's therapies. Sam and Kim thanked me often. Sam asked me once if I regretted spending money on therapies that did not produce desired results. I told him I regretted wasting money that could be spent more productively in other areas, but I would be more regretful if Kim came to me later and said Patrick would have been so much better if we had tried some therapy that we found unaffordable in earlier years.

I've often said, in the context of business, that any problem that can be solved with money is a good problem. For instance, if there is an auto accident and nobody is hurt, money will fix whatever damage the accident had caused. But if someone loses a limb or worse, no amount of money can make them whole again. No amount of money can make autism go away. I know how much this realization frustrates autism fathers, because men want go into the cave and develop a plan to fix it. First, identify the resources, find the money. But in this case, no amount of money can guarantee a fix for this ailment.

This fact hasn't slowed down the moms. I am constantly amazed at and gratified by the resourcefulness of autism moms. They have examined, tested, and evaluated every therapy, known and unknown, shared all of this on social media, and worked tirelessly to heal their children. Conventional medicine typically denies the value of this hard work because these autism moms don't have double blind studies by trained researchers with peer review and blue ribbons from the CDC, FDA, NIH, et al. The medical community wouldn't get a blue ribbon from me. They wouldn't even get a participation trophy. After the recently published statistic that one in forty-five children has autism, all the medical community can do is tell us it's not vaccines. That would be more believable if they could tell us what it is.

My daughter and many other autism moms believe vaccines are responsible for their children developing autism. I don't know if vaccines cause autism. I believe they do, but I don't know that they do. Here is what I do know, what is irrefutable. No other medication, protocol, therapy, or surgery in the field of medicine today comes without warning labels, list of possible negatives, percent of favorable outcome, etc. All of them do, except vaccines. If you are born in the morning, there is a good chance you will be vaccinated by dark, regardless of possible counterindications. If there's a history of immune deficiency in your family, shouldn't that be a consideration in the quantity and timing of vaccines? Will mumps, measles, and rubella return if children wait a few years for vaccinations, when maybe their immune systems are more developed?

After the shock of the diagnosis wears off, you go through the normal stages of denial, anger, resignation, etc. Unless you're the mother, in which case the anger never really goes away. The good news is that anger is an unbelievable motivator. My daughter Kim is relentless in her pursuit of the combination of treatments that will "cure" Patrick. The bad news is that anger is a heavy load to carry every day. It is like old age or gravity, working to wear you out twenty-four hours a day. You can't go anywhere to escape it. Even if everything and everybody responsible for your son's autism were extinguished from the Earth, it would not be enough to calm the anger inside.

Patrick is thirteen now. He is in the eighth grade with normal kids his age. He is happy more often than not. He shows genuine affection for his family members, including his grandparents, Nini and Pop. His primary interests are, first and foremost, movies, and then computers. If making a spreadsheet could bring world peace, he would be a Nobel Prize winner. His movie choices are well below age appropriate, but they are maturing over time. He has no interest in sports. Reading is a chore even with a subject matter he would be expected to embrace. When reading, he will ask what words mean. I spent several minutes with him one day explaining the dictionary before it dawned on me that he lives in a Google and debit card world. Dictionaries and cash need not apply.

I don't know whether I had a vision for him at thirteen when he was a baby. When Patrick was one or two, I remember staring at him playing and thinking of the summers he would spend with Nini and Pop. I would teach him how to be a champion golfer. We would go fishing and I would show him how to use a spinning reel, a bait caster, and a fly rod. He could know more than I about plastic lures, spinners, and jigs. All of those things are in my world; he's happier in his.

Patrick doesn't know he has autism. He's been told, but he doesn't really know. He went to his therapist recently, and upon returning, his dad asked him what they discussed. Patrick said, "We talked about worrying." Sam asked, "Well, is there something that worries you?" Patrick replied, "Yes, I'm afraid mom will not let me watch the *Jurassic Park* trilogy."

He is routinely coached to interact with others more appropriately because it is important to others. He seems completely unconcerned about his social awkwardness, except to the extent it displeases those close to him. He knows he is being asked to develop social skills (which are normally intuitive), and he wants to master those skills to please his parents and therapist, but not because it will make him more socially connected. That is, I've never heard him say he wants more friends or feels socially awkward. I can't say I've ever heard him engage in any introspection.

And yet, Patrick displays genuine affection, as opposed to a learned behavior that appears to be genuine affection. He seems also to be a born pleaser. He constantly receives praise from his teachers, and as a result of his desire to please, they have become big fans. As a result, he gets their best effort. All this effort has had incalculable effect on his progress, which, compared to others, has been extraordinary. Patrick is a model student who is always prepared for class. He feels responsibility for his assigned tasks; for instance, he takes care of his room without being reminded. He can also shake your hand, look you in the eye, and say, "My name is Patrick." This doesn't sound like much to a parent of neurotypical children, but to my family, WOW.

Somewhere back in time I thought Patrick was three, maybe four, years behind socially. Now I would say he and his support group have cut those three or four years in half. We have come from "distant and detached" to "a little nerdy," and we are well on our way to "confident and well mannered."

Pop
(Father of Team TMR's Blaze)

3

Shadow
Sunshine Lights the Way

STRENGTH DOES LIE IN NUMBERS. HAD THE THINKING MOMS NOT found each other, how would our kids possibly be able to deal with this autism journey? How would we, the grandparents, be able to deal with it, if not for our children and grandchildren showing us the way? Nothing could have prepared me for the last nine years. If someone had told me what my daughter's family would be dealing with, I wouldn't have believed them. My beautiful grandson having autism is, without question, the most emotionally painful thing imaginable. It reminds me of our air raid drills in the fifties. In these drills, we would duck and sit under our little desks, as if the bombs that we feared would somehow respect them.

What did we know? Until we got these grandkids, what did we know? I knew less than nothing. And knowing what I know now, I can't imagine how anyone could cope with this on their own. My daughter is the driver on this journey. My job is to assure her that she is going in the right direction and to marvel at how tenacious she is at finding this right direction. She has met this challenge head on, and she will win. I love her and would do anything for her, so I'm on board this bus rushing toward the recovery of this child that we both adore. It hasn't been pretty, and there is still a long way to go. But we are not alone, and neither are you. Find your support system and use it. Chances are that support system will be other people who are intimately familiar with autism. No one else has a clue.

I think of autism as a cruel sneak attack. You don't know when it will come or what it will bring. It drops into your life like a bomb and takes no prisoners. All autism families know when they first suspected and how it felt. They all have shared experiences. But this battle with autism is very personal, uniquely our own. Autism is sly and ever changing, like our own Rubik's cube from hell. This is the reality that our grandchildren, their parents, and the siblings face every day. With autism, one size does not fit all. We all have our stories to tell.

This is how I got here. My daughter, who is nicknamed Sunshine by the Thinking Moms, was, and still is, a person who takes charge of her life. She was sure of where she was going from the get-go, even as a young child. She was a delightful, easy kid to raise. It was almost like winning the kid lottery. Her dad and I would remark, "Where'd she come from?" I was in her shadow from the beginning, always watching, just in case she needed some guidance. This isn't as creepy as it sounds—that's what parents do. I was there if she should need me. She knew I was watching, and I think she's glad I was. Thankfully, I didn't need to step in often. She was always able to figure it out. She didn't take no for an answer. She knew how to find what would make her happy, work hard, play hard, and be a decent person. She did all the right things: college, graduate school, marriage to the man of her dreams. Their life was pretty close to perfect.

In 2003 she had, ta-da, this delicious baby boy, Rob. The first grandchild for both sets of grandparents, no less. He was perfect, just ask me. We grandparents became his second string minions, after mom and dad. The first year of Rob's life was what every parent expects: he was growing and developing, and he was so beautiful and engaging that it took my breath away. In Rob's second year, Sunshine began to notice subtle little things, the first signs of the A-bomb that would change our lives. She began searching online to see if she could find out what these subtle changes might be. During this time, she became pregnant with our second grandchild. Two years after Rob's birth, his brother, our equally delicious Quinn, was born. They weren't going to have the childhoods any of us had envisioned.

To this day, I'm not sure if anyone actually told my daughter that Rob had autism or if she figured it out herself. Denial in the beginning, I think, is necessary. How does one wrap their head around autism? Once autism enters your world, and you really learn what it is and what it can do, denial may be necessary for a while.

At first, I thought she'd just find a doctor who knew about this thing, autism, and they would guide her through it. He'd recover, and things would be hunky-dory, shouldn't take long, right? Okay, take a minute to chuckle. I was that naive. Despite receiving zero information about what autism was or how it could be fixed, my Sunshine became and continues to be relentless. She is the warrior and the advocate every child needs. She will not stop until Rob is recovered.

Maybe it's a good thing that we don't know what the future will bring. Learning what autism can do is almost beyond comprehension. No child, and I mean NO CHILD, should have to deal with this. No parent should see and feel what autism does to their child. As parents ourselves, we know that there is nothing worse than seeing our children hurting. This damn autism tries to take everything from them, and I mean everything. First it takes their beautiful children. Then it tries to ruin them, their health, marriage, relationships, and the wellbeing of their other children. And, hey, for good measure, let's bankrupt them too!

Families dealing with autism receive a personal Pandora's box filled with every imaginable emotion. Frighteningly so. How the hell are our children doing this? I mean, really, how do they get through the day? Day after day? It requires the kind of strength that only love can give them. These super-humans that are our children would go to the seventh circle of hell for their children, as we would for them. My job as Rob's grandparent is to love and support him without question or reservation. It's also my job to do the same for his parents and brother. They're the ones doing the heavy lifting here, day in, day out.

The thing that disturbs me the most is the emotional roller coaster that autism brings. Watching what happens—the good, the bad, and the ugly—and being helpless to help my own child, as she struggles to help hers. There have been many low points in the journey toward recovery. One brought us to our knees. When I think about that time and the emotional agony that my daughter and son-in-law went through, it almost seems unreal, like it was someone else's life.

At four years of age, Rob stopped growing. He wouldn't eat. Meal time was an ordeal, with Sunshine begging him to eat. Yes, begging him to eat. She said to me, "I can't even feed my child." The pain in her voice, the pain in her eyes, what could be said? She was desperate to find out what was happening and even more desperate to find a solution. This struggle over food went on for months and months. The little that Rob did eat was not being absorbed. He was so small for his age, and he was skin and bones. You've seen pictures of these children. I wish I were exaggerating here, but I'm not.

Sunshine was giving him supplements and searching for an answer, looking for someone who could help. Eventually she found a pediatric gastroenterologist who specialized in children with autism. The doctor suggested that Rob be scoped to see what might be going on in his gut. First he was given a capsule that was a pill cam. He wore a backpack with monitoring equipment for six hours, as the camera did its work recording what was going on in his gut. Next came the scope, for which he needed to be "cleaned out." You got it, enemas and laxatives. They worked. The next day Rob was scoped, and the doctors found that he had inflammation in his small intestine, similar to the inflammation caused by Crohn's disease. They also found that he had abnormal cells in his colon, which may have been signs of a previous inflammation. He was a trooper during these procedures, even though they must have been scary as hell for him.

That night, after Rob's mom slowly reintroduced food, he started to vomit. The doctor was contacted, and he said vomiting wasn't unusual in these situations. The vomiting continued, and the medication given to stop it didn't work. The next day, Rob began throwing up bile. He was taken to the emergency room and admitted to the hospital. Hospital personnel didn't think it was a result of being scoped because he wasn't throwing up blood. They weren't sure what was happening. I've learned that this statement is no surprise for autism parents. The doctors thought that maybe the pill cam hadn't passed. Rob was x-rayed, and the x-ray confirmed that the pill cam had passed. What it also showed was that there was a mass in his abdomen that looked like a blood clot. Thus began many more tests and procedures.

At this point, our Rob, who had been a rock star during this hellish process, had had enough. He refused to drink the barium—it's nasty stuff. This wonderful child, who had been through more than enough, had a tube inserted down his nose so the barium could get to his stomach. He was crying and begging them to stop. That was the point where my daughter nearly lost her mind; she wanted to kill the hospital personnel with her bare hands. My son-in-law sat sobbing. Rob would spend a week in the hospital. During that time, my daughter did not leave him, except to use the bathroom. The mass in his abdomen was getting smaller, so the doctors were confident it was a blood clot. They did not know where the blood clot had come from, but said it would resolve over time. Now they could get the GI problem fixed and get him to start gaining weight.

The next nine months were a hell of different medications prescribed for Rob's GI problem. They caused pain and excruciating headaches. He did not gain weight. The next step was supposed to be a medication that had the potential to alter his DNA and maybe cause cancer. It goes without saying that this was not an option.

Back to the research and looking for a doctor who might help. Sunshine found another DAN! doctor. He certainly didn't have all the answers, but he proved to be helpful, and the weight and growth came, ever so slowly. Rob is still small for his age and his gut issues are not 100 percent resolved, but his appetite has improved and he is eating healthy and organic food. Most importantly, he is here and with us. Given what he went through, I was at one point terrified that he wouldn't be.

I didn't share my fear and angst with her during that time. She had enough of those for all of us. She was working to take care of Rob and her family. My place is to be there for her and carry my own emotional baggage. That doesn't mean that my daughter doesn't want to hear how I feel; she does, she cares very much about my feelings. It's important to her that I be on board with her decisions. On more than one occasion she has said to me, "Do you think I'm crazy?" This is usually after she runs a new protocol or therapy by me, one that she thinks may be beneficial for Rob. My answer to that question is always "No." No one loves this kid more than she does. Who am I to second-guess the decisions she makes? She would never jeopardize his well-being. And yes, some of the things she's run by me seemed nuts. But what do I know? And who's to say whether they might work?

Sunshine and her family are into year nine of this autism trek. I am constantly amazed at their emotional toughness. She is determined to find recovery for Rob. She has that twenty-four hour a day job and still works at maintaining as "normal" as possible a life for her family. They are involved with their community and schools, and the boys are both involved in sports. Both she and her husband are the first people to lend a hand to anyone who may need help. Nothing ever seems to be too much to handle. I'm amazed at their physical toughness too. I worry for their health and am grateful that they work at keeping healthy.

All of the challenges just make them more determined. They will not allow themselves to cave in to autism. If they can be this strong, then I need to be strong. No second guessing. No saying, maybe you should do this, maybe you should do that, because guess what? They have already thought of it. Mom and Dad are always a step ahead of us.

If we look at life from the vantage point of what we lack, we won't see the good things we have. While autism is working to strip us of everything, we have to be working even harder to keep and grow what we do have. We need to keep our eyes on the prize, which is recovery for these kids. They deserve no less from us. Easy to say, not so easy to do. It's extraordinarily hard to stay positive. Autism brings some of the worst stuff in the world, and during those darkest times, survival in itself is a win. Where do our children find the strength and the resources to keep pushing? It's simple: they have no choice. Is there any one of us who hasn't had our own meltdown? You know, in a fetal position, sobbing, with snot coming out of your nose. Meltdowns may be keeping us sane. If you know how bad you can feel, you also know how great you can feel. Nothing can beat the feeling of seeing the gains our grandchildren make.

I can't talk about my personal experience with autism without including the entire family. It affects the whole family. My grandson's recovery will be because of his parents. I don't live with my daughter; we don't even live in the same state, and I need at least a three-hour heads-up to get there. I don't see all that they do and endure on a daily basis. What I do know is that they, like all families dealing with autism, are paying a huge price. It seems everyone gets the short straw.

Autism took from my grandson the person he was supposed to be. The fact that he is loved without question is not enough to make up for the fact that he didn't get his fair shot at childhood. And yes, that makes me angry. How miserably unfair. His brother, Quinn, didn't get his fair shot at his childhood either. These two beautiful boys should be laughing and carefree, conspiring like brothers do, putting one over on the parents. They should be talking about school and sports. Playing games, for God's sake. The big "A" has given them something totally different. They are very close and love each other dearly. Rob depends on Quinn as if he were a touchstone. That's a big responsibility for a nine-year-old, but our mighty Quinn handles it with maturity far beyond his years. He does have his moments, but he's only nine. And he needs to be heard as well—it can't be all autism. I can't say enough about the amazing siblings who are fighting this battle right beside their parents. Our Quinn is a kind, smart, compassionate person. Another kid lottery win for us. We love these kids like crazy.

Sunshine and her husband make a formidable team. My son-in-law is truly one of the best people I'll ever know. He's the guy you want your daughter to marry. Autism took their marriage and turned it in a direction they couldn't have foreseen; autism took Ozzie and Harriet and put them on the dark side of the moon. Sunshine and Jon tenaciously work at not allowing autism to take over their marriage. Marriage under the best of circumstances is hard work. Marriage and autism? Well, good luck. Too many date nights deferred, no candlelit dinners, no rose petals up the stairs. Some days you can give 90 percent and some days you can maybe muster .5 percent. It's those .5 percent days that require teamwork and knowing why you're together in the first place. One of my unending prayers is that my daughter and son-in-law keep their marriage strong. These kids will grow, and the situation will evolve and change. There has to be life after all this work, and they deserve that life.

So, is there anything good in all of this? Yes, it's what keeps us going. That box we received, the one with all the furies of hell . . . there was one other thing in that box. Pandora was a clever girl—she hid it at the bottom, so we had to look for it. This last thing to appear was the spirit of hope. Without hope, we would pack our tents and leave town. Hope is the motivator that we use in every aspect of our lives. Think about it. Hope I'm happy, win the game, get a better job, lose that weight, earn more money. This good stuff we hope for happens every day. And, I'd argue, it's because people not only hope but also work like hell to achieve their goals. Hope without the work is just hope. Hope combined with love and work can (and does) move mountains.

Rob is eleven now. He is not fully recovered, but that is on the way. My daughter and son-in-law have committed everything to that goal. What will my role be in his recovery? How do I try to support this family that I adore? Simple—I step back and watch. Sunshine knows she only needs to say the word and I'll step up. My promise to her was that we're in this together, no matter what. I learned long ago that when everything else falls away, what's left is family. One other thing I learned was that my children and grandchildren have given me more than I can ever give them. Kids make us better people, because they take us out of ourselves.

Bottom line is that always and forever, I've hitched my wagon to these semi-crazy people. Sunshine is driving this crazed autism bus, with her GPS set to recovery, no alternate routes. She doesn't take no for an answer. How this bus gets there is anyone's guess. It will be a bumpy ride. I'm a willing passenger, along with the rest of my wonderful family. Unending love and thanks go to the quieter family members (they know who they are). They keep the rest of us semi-grounded.

We will do more laughing than crying. We will prop each other up when needed. We will also let each other know when we're running off the rails. That's what family does, crazy or sane. In the end, Rob's story is for Sunshine, Jon, and Quinn to tell. But Rob proved to me what I had already thought was true: unconditional, almost maniacal love is all that matters in this world. My only and unending prayer now is that this family stays healthy and intact, and that they find the strength to reach their goals.

I don't need to look for heroes. I know who they are and where to find them.

Karen Doolan Sheibley
(Mother of Team TMR's Sunshine)

4

Gypsy

Autism Times Two—Clearing the Way for Hope and Healing

"IT'S OFFICIAL. JORDAN HAS AUTISM TOO . . ." "OH NO," I THOUGHT, as I read this text from my daughter Beth after my two-year-old grandson's evaluation. What could I possibly say that would make any difference at all? It had been devastating to learn, almost exactly a year earlier, that my granddaughter Olivia had been diagnosed with significant developmental and neurological delays attributed to autism. Now Jordan, too, was on the spectrum? Those words dealt a shot to my heart and my gut that was almost too much to bear—I could only imagine what Beth was feeling.

Olivia (we call her Livvie) was born in November 2009 after a high-risk pregnancy during which Beth had numerous ultrasounds to monitor the baby's growth. Beth had issues with her blood pressure throughout the pregnancy. As her due date drew near, her blood pressure rose to a dangerous level, so her doctor decided to induce labor four weeks early. Multiple doses of drugs designed to aid in inducing labor were given to my daughter, but Livvie was (and is!)

a stubborn little girl, so she clung tenaciously to her place in Beth's womb and ultimately had to be delivered by C-section. She was a tiny thing, and because her bilirubin level was low, she spent the first few days of her life in the neonatal nursery in an Isolette under the lamps, sporting her baby-sized goggles to protect her eyes from the light. When she came home, she weighed just over five pounds.

My children and I have always been very close, and when Livvie was born, my son and I were living together with Beth and her husband for economic reasons, as well as because I had been recently divorced. I was thrilled to be an everyday part of Livvie's newborn life and more than willing to be a hands-on grandma. When I was home from work and Beth was tired or busy, I fed Livvie, changed her, played with her, walked with her when she cried, and rocked her to sleep. I loved every second of it! Livvie and I really bonded, and I felt connected to her on a level that I used to say was "cosmic," as though we had belonged to each other in another lifetime. Livvie had beautiful dark eyes, lots of dark hair, and the sweetest dimpled smile I had ever seen. As you can probably tell, I was totally smitten with my granddaughter!

But there were also signs of trouble. As a baby, Livvie had trouble eating and sleeping. She would sometimes scream for hours as we paced the floor trying to soothe her. The pediatrician diagnosed Livvie with reflux disease when she was two months old, and she was given medication for that condition for several months. She also hated riding in the car. At the time, Beth was driving from Joliet, Illinois, to Gary, Indiana, every morning for her job, and Livvie would be dropped off close to my daughter's workplace to spend the day with her aunt while Mommy was at work. The long car ride was a killer, and Livvie was not a happy passenger. Eventually, Beth began to notice that certain music seemed to calm Livvie—she loved ABBA, of all things, especially the song "Dancing Queen"!

As Livvie grew, she was a bit slow to roll over, crawl, and walk, but she had that beautiful smile and lots of attitude, and I was sure that she would meet every milestone in her own time. By eight months, she was waving, saying "dada," and sitting up on her own. She finally began rolling over at will when she was around nine months old. We have lots of photos of Livvie around that age that show her smiling, and laughing, and flashing her dimples.

As she neared the age of twelve months, however, something about Livvie seemed to change. She became more withdrawn and babbled less. She didn't want to be around people. During a large family party for Livvie's first birthday, she was unusually silent and seemed uncomfortable with all the noise and activity. She wouldn't say any of her words or wave bye-bye to any of her relatives. For the most part, this state of silence and withdrawal persisted over the next several months. There were still some smiles, but they were much fewer, and Livvie no longer seemed at ease in her world. She finally learned to walk at around fourteen months, but the babbling had virtually disappeared.

When Livvie still did not have any basic language at eighteen months, Beth began to become concerned. Her pediatrician agreed that something was amiss, and Livvie began receiving early intervention in the form of speech, occupational, and developmental therapy multiple times every week. Speech therapy was meant to help Livvie learn how to form and express her words, as well as how to understand the words that were spoken to her and listen and respond to verbal cues. Developmental therapy helped monitor all aspects of Livvie's development, such as speech, cognitive skills, gross and fine motor skills, and sensory processing, in order to help close the developmental gaps and get her ready for school. Occupational therapy helped Livvie learn various life skills appropriate for her age, like dressing herself, brushing her teeth, and most importantly, how to play imaginatively—something with which many children with autism have a very difficult time.

One thing that hadn't changed during all this time was Livvie's love of music. She had become obsessed with a Nickelodeon program called *The Fresh Beat Band*. At one point, we had more than fifty episodes of the show on our DVR, and Livvie wanted the show on all day, every day. Her love of the show was used as a motivational tool for the therapists, a way to get Livvie to cooperate with their requests in order to earn a few minutes of watching *The Fresh Beat Band*.

When Livvie was around ten months old, Beth became pregnant again. It was another high-risk pregnancy, with similar issues as the ones Beth experienced while pregnant with Livvie. Since Livvie had been born by C-section, Jordan's birth would be a scheduled Caesarian delivery as well. When Beth was approximately six weeks from Jordan's due date, her amniotic fluid dropped below what her doctor considered a safe level, and she was hospitalized and given drugs to help the baby's lungs mature prior to delivery. My grandson Jordan was born six weeks premature on March 21, 2011. Even though he was premature, Jordan was at a healthy birth weight and had none of the issues Livvie experienced in her first few days of life.

Shortly after Livvie's second birthday, we hosted our extended family for Thanksgiving. As soon as relatives began to arrive, Livvie started to scream uncontrollably, and we could only get her to calm down by taking her to another room, where one of us (Beth, her husband, or I) had to hold her and watch *The Fresh Beat Band* with her. That was the last family party we hosted to this day. Two months later, Livvie had a formal evaluation and was determined to be delayed in almost every aspect of her development. We received the devastating diagnosis that she had autism.

The weeks after Livvie's diagnosis were really difficult for our family. You don't realize all the hopes, and dreams, and expectations that take root in your mind and heart when a child or grandchild is born until they're all dashed away in the instant you hear the word "autism." What would Livvie's future hold now? Would she ever be able to tell us what she was feeling or thinking? Would she ever dance in a recital or play a sport? Would she ever go to a homecoming dance or to prom? Would she ever fall in love, get married, have her own beautiful babies? Would she ever even be self-sufficient enough to live on her own and support herself? I was worried and heartbroken for my granddaughter, and I knew that Beth was suffering terribly as a result of Livvie's diagnosis. For her sake, I refused to give in to all the dark thoughts and struggled to find the hope and optimism that were in my nature. I wanted to be there for both my daughter and my granddaughter in whatever way they needed me.

Meanwhile, Jordan seemed to be growing and thriving. He was walking at nine months and didn't seem to be experiencing any of the food issues that Livvie had. He did have some quirky behaviors and a bit of trouble controlling his emotions, and he also was somewhat slow to talk, but many boys develop language a bit later than girls. Because Jordan was not communicating much verbally by eighteen months, he also began receiving early intervention therapies at that age. Just before his second birthday, Jordan also received a diagnosis of autism.

Though Jordan was clearly higher functioning than Livvie, the fact that both of our babies were on the spectrum was shattering. I had no idea what I could possibly say that would provide any comfort to Beth, other than reassure her that Livvie and Jordan were lucky to have been born to the absolute best mom they could hope for—one who I knew would search tirelessly for ways to help her children recover from this insidious disease.

By the time of Jordan's diagnosis, Livvie and Jordan were both using iPads, both as educational tools and for entertainment. Jordan was very focused on letters and numbers and would watch numerous videos and play games related to basic letter introduction. Around the time he was nineteen or twenty months old, Jordan could spell a variety of words. By his second birthday, when he finally began talking, we realized that he had taught himself to read! We were amazed, to say the least. Jordan would watch videos about letters on the iPad all day; soon, he could recite the alphabet. He quickly learned to spell words like "imagination," "environment," and "conscientious"—words that were way beyond the capabilities of most two-year-olds. He could also sound out words and read books meant for first-graders. For months, we bought him every alphabet puzzle and game we could find, and Jordan continued to astound us with his reading and spelling skills. He even taught himself sign language!

Beth, trusting her intuition, began researching this self-taught reading ability and discovered a condition called hyperlexia, defined as a syndrome characterized by an intense fascination with letters or numbers and an advanced reading ability. Often, hyperlexia and autism spectrum disorder go hand-in-hand. Unfortunately, even though children with hyperlexia exhibit advanced word skills, they often have no comprehension of the words that they read. Beth's conclusion that Jordan had hyperlexia was eventually confirmed by his developmental pediatrician.

When Livvie was diagnosed with autism, Beth began talking to all the therapists, conducting research on the Internet, and reading all kinds of materials about ASD. She learned that many kids on the spectrum have digestive issues that can be improved or resolved by gluten- and casein-free diets. After a bit of trial and error, Livvie's diet became dairy-free when she was around two and a half years old, and she began to sleep through the night for the first time ever!

Beth also learned about all the chemicals we were unknowingly being exposed to and ingesting every day, and we began to consciously try to eliminate some of those chemicals by eating organic and non-GMO foods and choosing more natural or organic household products whenever possible. To be honest, I was very disturbed to realize that I had never really thought about the chemicals I put into or onto my body every day. Hair products, cosmetics, soaps and body lotions, air fresheners, laundry and cleaning products, processed foods, dairy products, beef, chicken, fruits, and vegetables all either contained or were being treated with a number of harmful chemicals. Yikes! This was truly a wake-up call . . . no more going through life in the bliss of ignorance. I began to carefully study product labels, read articles, and follow blogs, looking for safer alternatives to the products we had been using for years.

In the meantime, the kids got older. In Illinois, where we live, kids age out of the Early Intervention System when they turn three. At that point, the parent can enroll the child in the local school system or choose alternative therapy sources. Livvie started school shortly after turning three. As a result of the school's evaluation and Beth's meeting with school authorities to put Livvie's individualized education plan (IEP) in place, Livvie was placed in a class for special needs children, specifically for those with autism. The class enrollment was limited to eight children, and each child had an individual aide working with them at all times.

Beth could have sent Livvie to school full time, but because she was very worried about Livvie's reaction to a strange new environment and the separation from her, Beth elected to start Livvie off on a part-time basis. As Beth had feared, the transition was very difficult for Livvie, and consequently for Beth. Livvie often cried and screamed, kicked, and pushed to avoid being buckled into her car seat on the bus. Things weren't much better when she arrived at school.

Luckily, Livvie became attached to one of her aides, and positive reinforcement in the way of *Fresh Beat Band* videos eventually helped her settle into the new routine of school attendance. Livvie's detachment, or her retreat to what was called her "autism bubble," persisted even after she started school. She also remained largely nonverbal. Many times I looked at pictures of Livvie from earlier days and felt so very sad, wondering if our beautiful smiling Olivia would ever come back to us. I repeatedly watched a treasured video of Livvie where she is standing with her hand on her hip and giving us a lecture in her Livvie-babble, so full of the attitude and personality I knew were still somewhere inside her. I missed her desperately.

Jordan also started school when he turned three; no surprise to us, his evaluation and IEP resulted in his being placed in a class for special needs children who are not as severely affected by their diagnoses or disabilities. There is one aide for every five children, and this class is part time by design. Because of Jordan's hyperlexia, Beth made sure that part of his education focuses on word comprehension and context so that he does not fall behind his peers in these areas. For the most part, Jordan has thrived in school, since he loves to learn so much that it makes up for the fact that his reading and spelling skills are quite a bit ahead of his classmates and he is quite often being taught things that he already knows. He has continued to receive speech and occupational therapy outside of school, as has Livvie, and Jordan's conversational and receptive language skills are improving all the time. Jordan's ability to control his emotions remains his greatest challenge at this point. He will frequently see or hear something that causes him to burst into tears for no reason that is apparent even to him and will ask for help calming down. He also gets very upset when he's watching a video on the iPad and an ad pops up or he's playing a game and it doesn't progress the way he anticipates. Jordan's emotional reaction to these and other situations is far more intense than that of the average child, but he is still very young and has lots of time for improvement.

Based on her research and the recommendations from some of her friends whose children were also on the spectrum, Beth began a homeopathic treatment for Livvie and Jordan called CEASE during the summer of 2013, when Livvie was three and a half and Jordan was twenty-seven months old. Homeopathic remedies for various "injuries" stemming from the vaccinations the kids had received and the many ultrasounds and drugs administered to Beth during her pregnancies were prescribed and given to Livvie and Jordan several times per week for a number of weeks. They also took supporting supplements on certain of the off-days from the remedies. Each treatment was called a "clear," and the process would sometimes lead to physical symptoms, such as a fever or a rash, or emotional or psychological ones. Occasionally, there were no discernible side effects from the clears whatsoever.

The clears followed a schedule prescribed by the homeopath. They began with clearing the medications Beth received for her blood pressure during her pregnancies, followed by a clear for the drugs she was given to induce labor. We noticed small improvements in the kids' language and behavior after these clears, but nothing like we were hoping for. Next, the homeopath began prescribing clears for certain of the vaccinations that Liv and Jordan had received before their ASD diagnoses. When the kids received the clear for the hepatitis B vaccine, the effects on Livvie were astonishing! She started vocalizing many more words each day, and while she did not pronounce them perfectly, the word approximations were now so much clearer and more understandable. In addition, Livvie began to emerge from the autism bubble—she seemed more aware of her surroundings, she began to interact more with us, and she just seemed to bloom. She flashed her beautiful dimpled smile much more frequently, and those big brown eyes were full of life and mischief again. There are few things in life I have ever felt more grateful for!

Some subsequent clears have brought more subtle improvements for Livvie, but I am very thankful for every small gain. It has been more difficult to see any substantive gains from the clears for Jordan, since he is already so good with words and language and has always been very expressive with his emotions. I believe that the clears have helped him achieve some of the significant improvements he has made with his expressive (getting words out) and receptive (understanding what he hears) language, and we are hopeful that we will continue to see more positive results.

One of the more surprising and disturbing things I have learned from my daughter concerns the safety and efficacy of today's vaccines. I was somewhat reluctant to believe that vaccines could have contributed to or been a cause of autism in any child; after all, both of my kids and all of my nieces and nephews had been vaccinated without any negative repercussions. I was completely unaware that so many more vaccines had been added to the recommended schedule of vaccinations and that toxic substances were being used to bind them together. I began to read stories and blogs by the moms and dads in the TMR community and others chronicling the changes and regressions their children experienced after receiving certain vaccinations. And I began to feel concerned. Why were infants who had barely taken their first breaths being vaccinated against a sexually transmitted disease? Why did any child need to receive nine or ten or a dozen vaccinations at once? Why did the vaccine contain toxic chemicals? Why would the CDC refuse to investigate in any meaningful way whether vaccines had any culpability in the ever-growing numbers of children being diagnosed with ASD every year?

When I began to believe that the answers to these questions could all be traced back to the unsavory relationship between major pharmaceutical companies and the government agencies we rely upon to ensure the safety of vaccines for our children, I began to feel more than concerned—I began to feel outraged! The more I read and learn, the more I advocate awareness and fully informed choices for every parent who considers vaccinating their child. I also advocate a parent's choice to refuse certain or all vaccinations and/or adopt a more reasonable schedule of vaccinations for their child. I believe that until the CDC and other government agencies are barred from allowing representatives of the companies whose products they are tasked with regulating to hold offices or participate in their regulatory processes, none of our children will be safe from the potential dangers of current vaccines.

Being a grandparent to two children with autism is both challenging and rewarding, as I'm certain must be the case with any disease or disability. In order to ensure that Beth can be a stay-at-home mom with Livvie and Jordan, which has been necessary to manage their school and therapy schedules (and because daycare, and particularly daycare for special needs children, is prohibitively expensive), I have continued to work a sometimes demanding and stressful job in order to help support our family. For now, I have had to put aside any thoughts of imminent retirement, as well as my plans to save a substantial sum of money while I am still making a good income. In the next few years, I will probably further deplete my retirement funds to help purchase a permanent home in a school district that is good for special needs children. Honestly, though, those are the least of my concerns.

Instead, I worry about what will happen to my grandchildren as they grow up. There is hope that Jordan will eventually lose his autism diagnosis and be mainstreamed in school, but that change will not come without consequences. Children can be cruel, and I worry that his quirky personality and the fact that he wears his emotions on his sleeve might make him the subject of jokes, humiliation, and possibly bullying. I worry that Livvie, as a female, might be frightened of the changes that will happen to her body as she grows older and may fall prey to those that will take advantage of and exploit her innocence. Livvie can also be aggressive with Beth sometimes, and I worry that Beth might be unable to manage Livvie's aggression as she grows older and stronger. I ask myself what will happen to my family when I pass on, and what will happen to Livvie and Jordan when they are eventually left alone in this world without me or their parents.

I know that Beth and her husband worry about these things too. It hurts my heart that my daughter's life will never be "normal" in the sense that the lives of parents with typical children are. I'm sad that she may have to spend every day of her life worrying about the effects and consequences that autism is having on her children. So because I love Beth and my grandchildren with everything I am, I try, when I can, to shoulder some of the load and provide a few hours' respite from the worry and challenges they face every day.

My reward is watching my daughter and her husband raise these two beautiful kids with love, and strength, and grace every single day. My reward is having a front-row seat to the growth, and gains, and achievements of these two beautiful little people and knowing that I've contributed to them in some small way. My reward is the smiles, the hugs, and the "Hi, Grandma" I get when I come home from work. My reward is knowing that autism hasn't beaten us and that it never will.

Kathleen Pritchard
(Friend of Team TMR)

5

Team Hudson
A Journey Paved in Love

FOR MY WIFE LORI AND ME, GRANDPARENTING HAS TRULY BEEN A rewarding and enjoyable experience. It's like getting a second chance at being a parent, only this time you're more prepared, armed with knowledge, experience, and stability. What could go wrong?

Enter autism.

The enjoyable and rewarding parts still hold true, but whatever knowledge or experience you thought you had probably goes right out the door. Terms like "spectrum," "vaccine injury," "protocol," "regression," and "biomed"—things that we had heard very little of before— are now commonplace lingo. The daughter that we raised and taught on her way to adulthood has now found herself having to educate us on the new terminology and its meanings. We have learned a lot but definitely have a whole lot more to absorb, and the learning process has left us amazed, proud, and heartbroken all at the same time.

Our first experience in grandparenting took us by surprise. Our daughter became pregnant at a young age. We welcomed Bailey, our first grandchild, into our lives with love and hope. We were just so glad that he was healthy. The timing may not have been what we expected, but looking back, it was an era that we would not change for the world.

It was almost twelve years later that Hudson, our second grandson, arrived. Our daughter Amanda and her husband Justin were happily married and building a home, with great anticipation of Hudson's arrival. Everything seemed to be just the way we would have written in a script, as another healthy and thriving baby boy was born. Knowing how much we enjoy Bailey, we knew the addition of another grandchild, Hudson, would be a wonderful experience for us all. He has taken center stage in our lives for nearly five years.

At the same time, however, due to vaccine injury that he received at six months and a subsequent injury at fifteen months that caused immediate regression, the demands of parenting and grandparenting have been greatly intensified. Autism doesn't just affect your grandchild; it affects the entire family. To deal with it, we have become Team Hudson.

Our daughter Amanda has become a full-fledged warrior mom who spends the majority of her available time researching, mentoring, and reacting to all things autism. Words cannot describe just how proud we are of her. She is relentless in her quest to remedy the situation that her tiny "H-Man" has been dealt. She has also helped countless other warrior moms and dads with finding menu and therapy options, as well as with navigating their child's many medically complex conditions and organizing fundraising efforts to fight their battle. We are proud of the amazing autism advocate that she has become and the fact that she does not limit her knowledge to just parents affected by vaccine injury—she also helps to educate and assist other moms in making informed decisions for their families.

Unfortunately, this constant struggle does take its toll on her. Fortunately, her husband Justin is a very helpful and compassionate partner. Because he is a wonderful provider, he has allowed Amanda to concentrate her efforts entirely on the task at hand without the additional burden of having to be employed as well. She is on call 24/7, but when Justin gets home, he does a great job of helping with Hudson's care in a passionate and unselfish manner. We are extremely proud of him as well.

Big brother Bailey is also a vital member of Team Hudson. There is no one whom Hudson admires more in this world than his big "brudder." They love each other and play well together. However, being the popular, athletic, and socially active teen that he is, Bailey sometimes has limited time for his baby brother.

And what about us, the grandparents? Perhaps the biggest struggle we face as grandparents of a child with autism is the fact that we don't completely know what to do to help. Sure, we can help financially with therapies, doctors, or protocol expenses. We can also babysit every now and then to give Amanda and Justin a break, but we wish we could perform some type of magic that would suddenly make Hudson become verbal and free of pain. Instead, we must use notes from Amanda stating what to feed him and when, what supplements to administer, and what essential oils should be applied where and when.

Hudson is usually a good boy at Gran's house, and he sleeps through the night on his occasional sleepovers that we look forward to. But we have also witnessed some heartbreaking meltdowns. I recall one recent episode where he was, as Amanda describes it, trying to get out of his own skin. Watching him run around in panic mode where nothing seemed to provide relief, not even his beloved swimming pool, was almost unbearable.

I prayed for God to transfer the pain to me instead of that innocent little boy, and when that didn't work, I angrily shot the finger to the heavens. (An act I regret and have asked forgiveness for every day since.)

There are better ways to cope. All of our family members have been affected by the struggles brought on by autism, and we all

accept and deal with them in our own ways. My daughter is relentless with her research, as well as mentoring and sharing with others
on her social media groups. Her husband understands how taxing
her days can be, so he enjoys helping take over Hudson's care with
some quality time of their own, be it playtime, bath time, or whatever happens along. In my case, I have found that writing serves as a
sort of therapy and helps me process life events, so I am including a
poem I wrote a few years back:

The Puzzle

Autism
It's just a word
It doesn't affect me
That's absurd
If that's your stance
For you, that's great
You must not know
That 1 out of 88
But if you do
You know it's real
And dealing with it
Is quite an ordeal
Hudson, my grandson
Is just 2 years old
And if was able to speak
What stories could be told
Does he know who I am?
Does he know his own name?
Will he make his own friends?
Will he join in on a game?
What is happening in his head?
I'd sure like to know
Does he realize he's the luckiest

Little man I know?
His Mom is a Warrior
Who goes to battle each day
Developing a plan of attack
Fighting for him the whole way
His father's and brother's support
Just can't be beat
As they adapt to his schedule
And change what they eat
Yes, Hudson's affliction
Has brought changes for sure
It's taught patience and compassion
As we strive for a cure
The Autism puzzle
Is a difficult circumstance
But Team Hudson is there
To give him his best chance
Will he improve, or stay the same
It's too early to say
But he will be cherished and loved
Every step of the way!!!

It pains me to realize that autism numbers have increased so much in the two short years since this poem was written. Based on studies of twelve-year-olds, a demographic my grandson is not even included in, the autism rate is now underreported at one in forty-five.

Fortunately, the enjoyable experiences we have had in helping raise our grandson far outweigh the painful ones, and we realize how blessed we are to have this little guy in our lives. We know that things certainly could be worse, and we are extremely grateful that they are not.

The perception of having a child with autism in the family is that it is terrible in all aspects, but the reality is that there are countless examples of how it can be an enriching and rewarding experience.

Small achievements, such as making eye contact or showing off "super fancy" tumbling tricks, may go unnoticed or unappreciated from a typically functioning child, but are cherished and celebrated immensely in our family. This is because every milestone reached, big or small, is fought for 100 times harder. Every milestone reached is such a thrill to experience, and each leaves us with anticipation and desire to reach the next step in his progress. We also accept that he might not make any further progress and know that he is still a huge blessing and tremendous source of richness in our lives. Hudson's giggle and million-dollar smile bring joy to everyone he meets. And for that we are truly grateful.

These children are true warriors, and we have learned more from them than we could ever teach them. In addition to becoming more aware and learning about things like nutrition, supplements, and therapies, we have also become better at virtues like love, nurturing, and patience—all as a result of being involved in our grandson's upbringing.

One thing we know for sure is that there has been no shortage of love and pride in our journey with Hudson.

God's blessings to you all,

David and Lori Findley
(Friends of Team TMR)

6

Guamma
My Hero

I DON'T WANT TO WRITE THIS!!! THERE, I SAID IT. I AM NOT A WRITER, and I have certainly never considered myself a thinker. I am a mother, grandmother, aunt, sister, and friend. I am doing this because of my daughter, Laura, and my grandson, Trevor. I want their story to be told. My hope in writing this is that I can give hope and inspiration to other grandparents who might read my story.

I have not always been a thinking grandparent. Like many of you, I grew up in the baby boomer generation, where we were taught to follow the rules and doctors' orders. I have five children, and I taught them to follow the rules as well.

But all the rules changed when my grandson Trevor regressed into autism. I now question things that I never would have questioned before. I do things that I never would have done before. I have stepped way outside of my comfort zone and realized that a lot of what I believed and had been taught my whole life is not true. I was naïve and trusted everyone. Not anymore.

Life isn't always fair. We do not always get to live it the way we would like to or had planned to, but we make the most of it and go on. We do our best to make the lives of our loved ones as happy and fulfilled as we can. This is what has happened in my family. We are here to help and guide Trevor as best we can. We love him and want to see him succeed. It is my daughter's knowledge that has gotten my grandson to the level he is at right now; my role has been to support her by being her sounding board, friend, and mother. I listen and console, and I am there for her when she needs me. She is my life, and I love her for all that she does for everyone.

I have had the unusual experience of being able live with my daughter and her family since her first child, Trevor, was born. I was living in a different state when she got pregnant, but my daughter and her husband asked me to come and live with them in California to help with their son after his birth. My daughter was going back to work full time, and they did not want to put their son in daycare. I moved in with them six weeks before Trevor was born and ended up staying for the past seventeen years.

I loved the time I got to spend watching Trevor develop and grow into a little boy. My daughter worked five days a week, so at that time I was with him more than she was. We developed an incredible bond. He started walking and talking early. He hit all of his milestones earlier than what the medical profession says is standard. He rolled over, sat up, babbled, played peek-a-boo, laughed, pointed, crawled, walked, and talked, all ahead of schedule. I was present at all of his well-child visits and remember how impressed the doctor was with him and how advanced he was. He was a gorgeous, happy, and loving little boy.

When the time came for Trevor to get his required immunizations, Laura asked me what I thought about them. I told her that I had all her brothers and sister immunized and that none of them had any problems, so I saw nothing wrong with her having her son get his shots. Little did I know that the number of shots had increased drastically between then and now, and that the ingredients in the shots had changed as well. Laura's in-laws did not vaccinate for religious reasons, so she was torn. Being the good girl I taught her to be, she followed the rules, did what the doctor ordered, and had her son injected with what would cause the beginning of his regression into autism.

Shortly after Trevor received his MMR vaccine (and others) at the young age of around twelve months, his world—as well as ours—began to change. He withdrew into himself and has never been the same since. The child who used to be my beautiful, happy grandson was now someone who did not talk much or make eye contact with anyone. He was in his own little world, and we did not know how to enter it.

Even before the official diagnosis of autism, Trevor began to change dramatically. He would line up all of his Matchbox cars in a straight line—and I mean straight, perfectly straight. If any car did not line up and touch, he would get upset and adjust it until it did. He had a lot of cars, and they were lined up all over the house. Then he started adding other items into the lineup; they all had to match as well.

His communication patterns were also changing. Previously, when he wanted something, he was able to ask for it. Now he would take you by your hand and guide you to what he wanted and put your hand on it or near it, leaving you to guess what it was he wanted. Needless to say, a lot of times we couldn't figure it out, which led to frustration and tears.

He did not pay any attention to us when we talked to him. He just continued doing what he was doing, as though no one had spoken to him. He stopped responding to his name. He stopped taking naps, and we had to drive him around in the car to get him to sleep during the day. He seemed to be sick a lot and was put on a lot of antibiotics. When he was two, we took him to Disneyland, and he freaked out on the tram ride from the parking lot and didn't want to go on any of the rides. Laura and her friend went on rides, while I pushed Trevor in his stroller. What kid doesn't love Disneyland? It was clear that his entire world had changed.

Trevor also started to display other odd behaviors. He had to have something in his hand at all times and would proceed to look at what he was holding very closely. He would wiggle it back and forth in front of his eye. He also used to do what we called "hand puppets" with his fingers and then look at his fingers out of the corner of his eye. He started humming a lot. This, we thought, was Trevor being Trevor, but we did not see the big picture. Loud noises bothered him a lot, so he would always have his hands covering his ears in order to block everything and everyone out. He started to walk on his tiptoes. He would not walk in the grass with bare feet. We did not know at the time that these behaviors are associated with autism.

When Laura took Trevor in for his third-year checkup with the pediatrician, she was given the life-changing recommendation that she should have her son evaluated for autism. The doctor said that autism could be the reason for Trevor's strange behaviors and loss of skills. Since we had never encountered any children with autism or read anything on the subject, we never thought that this was his problem; we thought that these changes just had to do with who he was. We had no guidelines to follow and no one to talk to at this time. Needless to say, we were all in for a life-changing experience.

Laura was devastated and terrified. She had Trevor evaluated (on 9/11, of all days), and her pediatrician's suspicions were confirmed. Trevor was placed into a preschool program for "developmentally delayed" children. "Developmental delay" was what autism was called at the time. When Trevor was almost four years old, we moved from California to Nevada, and he was enrolled in another school program for "developmentally delayed" children. He went to school full time and had a lot of outside activities to help him. Meanwhile, Laura began spending countless hours exploring the Internet, reading books, listening to other parents who are experiencing the same difficulties, and doing everything possible to help her son.

It was excruciating to see the anguish and pain that my daughter endured. She had been handed the biggest challenge of her life. There was nothing I could do to take away her pain, but I could be there for her in any capacity that was needed. It is so hard to hear your child, no matter how old they are, cry with such pain. I am so thankful that she is such a strong person—the strongest I know.

This was not the first time that I had seen my daughter in such pain. Three years before Trevor was born, Laura was widowed. Her first husband, my beloved son-in-law, was killed in a car accident, and her world was turned upside down. I had to watch her suffer then too. I stayed with her for a while and helped her with anything she needed. At that time, she had no children, so it was just her (and her dog) that I was taking care of. What happened with Trevor was a different kind of suffering because this time it was her baby. No one should have to go through so much in their lifetime. No one.

Laura had to endure one more tragedy in her life a couple of years after we moved to Nevada. As is the case for many families who have children with autism, she and her husband got divorced. Again her world was turned upside down. I needed to step in and take the part of "daddy." I needed to be there even more now for this broken family. They were divorced for three years, got back together and were remarried for six more years, and then divorced again this year (2015). I am still living with Laura and her two boys, doing what I can to help her deal with the overwhelming stress that having a child with autism has placed on her.

She is now a full-time single mother to two teen boys, one with autism and one typical child (a straight-A student). She also works a couple of jobs. She is an author, editor, and a publisher. Her plate is overflowing, but she still spends any extra time she has finding more help for Trevor. Who could ask for a more dedicated mother? No one. She is amazing!

I usually do not question what she does. If I have any question about why she is doing something, I ask and she explains. I may not always agree, but I am here to back her up. When it comes to healing Trevor, I learned that my place was not to question her decisions but to abide by them. She is Trevor's mother, and she knows more than I do. She is the person that spends endless hours researching the ways to help her child.

In her search for answers, Laura discovered that Trevor had a lot of allergies and other health issues. Trevor's regular pediatrician was of no help, so Laura turned to alternative medicine. She talked to a lot of people who had success themselves in this matter, so she decided to try their recommendations with Trevor. She changed his diet. He was put on a gluten-free, casein-free diet. At the time, there were fewer such products available than there are today. My daughter made most of Trevor's food from scratch, without boxed mixes or pre-made food.

There was a lot of trial and error, and there were some disasters, but there was also a lot of good food. Trevor improved tremendously with this new diet. He was not always happy that he couldn't have what he used to eat, but he did eventually come to enjoy his new food. Laura removed everything with wheat in it. She learned to read the food labels. She had his food allergies and environmental allergies treated with an acupuncture (acupressure in children) technique called NAET.

These days Trevor eats a lot of fruit and vegetables. He always has the healthiest lunch at his school. He does eat some junk food, but it is organic and non-GMO. He is growing, so he eats all the time. He used to wait for someone to get his food, but now he helps himself to what he wants, when he wants it. To help him adjust, we have all changed our diets to match his so that there is no food that he should not eat lying around. His current favorite food is his gluten-free pizza. (I actually lost twenty pounds just by going gluten-free myself!)

But diet is not the only part of my life that has changed. There is a lot I have learned from Trevor. The biggest lesson is patience. I do not always have the patience I wish I had, but when I look into the face of this innocent young man, I step back, take a deep breath, and start all over again. His love and his need for my help take priority in my life.

My grandson is my hero! He never complains (almost never) and usually does what you ask him to do. He has to work harder and longer than most kids his age to learn and accomplish what is asked of him. He goes to school and has tutors that come to the house to work extra hours with him. His mother also works with him daily. He is always trying to achieve more and more tasks and learn more information.

His biggest obstacle to overcome has been regaining his speech. There was a time in his life when we were not sure that he would ever talk again. He understands what you say to him, but he struggles with his communication, though he can now ask for the things he wants to eat or do. He can read, write, do math, and type. He is becoming more and more independent—he likes to do things on his own that we used to do for him. He helps us with chores and likes to be involved with family activities.

And Trevor really loves his family. He has become a very affectionate young man. He gives hugs and kisses to people he knows. This wasn't always the case. When he was first diagnosed with autism, he often avoided physical contact. All this has changed, and I am loving it. Trevor improves daily, and my biggest hope is to see him recover.

My grandson and I still have a strong bond. He loves to hang out in my bedroom with me, either using my computer or watching his videos on my TV. We laugh, and giggle, and just hang out.

Every day I look at Trevor, I see all that he has accomplished, and I couldn't be more proud. Every day I am thankful to be a part of his life. I have watched him grow from a happy typical little boy into a happy young man. To be sure, there have been a lot of struggles along the way, and there is still a lot that needs to be done to get Trevor to where he needs to be. Through all of this, he has made me very proud to be his Guamma.

I chose the name "Guamma" for my nickname because this is what Trevor used to call me when he first started talking. He couldn't say "Grandma," so instead he called me "Guamma." This name holds a special meaning because it was his way of talking to *just me*. We usually tried to get him to correct his words, but this was the one that I wanted him to say the way he did. He now calls me "Grandma," but I miss him calling me "Guamma" and saying "I luff you Guamma."

When I look back on all that has happened in my life over the past seventeen years, one of the highlights is Trevor's smile. He has a million-dollar smile that lights up the room. He will always hold a special place in my heart. His hugs and kisses make me feel overjoyed with love.

My experience with Trevor also led me to begin working with other kids with special needs. For the past six years, I have also worked in a before-school and after-school program with the local Parks and Rec for elementary-school children. I started working with Trevor in this program, and when he stopped going there, my supervisor asked me if I would be willing to work with other special needs children. Because I love kids and want to help them in any way I can, I had to say yes. I have worked with other children with autism, a boy with cerebral palsy, and numerous boys and girls with other difficulties. These children need help to get by in our world they don't always understand. They need love and understanding. I learned a lot from them and from my grandson, and I am grateful for that.

But the struggles also continue and are all too real. The hardest part for me during Trevor's struggle with autism has been witnessing him having multiple grand mal seizures within the past two years. (He never had one before age fifteen.) He had the first one during one of his tutoring sessions. Luckily, his tutor had seen seizures in other children she worked with and was right there to help Trevor when it happened; I was in the other room and mom and dad were both at work. This seizure was the hardest on him and lasted the longest.

Fortunately, I have taken first aid and CPR classes, so I was able to help him and be there to comfort him. Dad and I were there during the second seizure. Dad was in the bathtub when it started, so he didn't see it, but I was there to protect and comfort him. Dad got out of the tub, picked Trevor up, and put him in his bed until the episode was over. During the next two, mom and dad were home. We all talked to Trevor, and I held his head and stroked his hair until the shaking stopped. He often bit his tongue and I had to clean up blood afterward. Each of his seizures was less severe, and he came around in less time. But talk about feeling helpless! Even though I knew what to do, I could not take the pain or suffering away from him. I am just thankful that I was there to help. And soon, just like she always does, my daughter figured out what was causing the seizures and took steps to prevent them from happening again.

The older Trevor gets, the more I worry about his future. These kids do grow up, and they continue to need a lot of support. The grandparents aren't getting any younger, either. I think that it is time for all grandparents of children with autism to pull together and stand up for our grandchildren's rights to secure supports for their future. We need to be there to be their voice in what happens to them, as well as to guide and protect them. What will happen to them if mom, and dad, and grandma are no longer here? We need to have safe alternative living arrangements for them. We can't expect that their siblings or other family members will take care of them. There is much work to be done. With the autism rate skyrocketing, the situation is only going to get worse. There are already waiting lists for everything and a shortage of providers.

Most of our children are not doctors, but they literally have had to become doctors, and they are doing the best they can to help their kids. They sometimes struggle, and we need to be supportive of them. We need to let them know we love them and will always be there for them. This is our role in their lives. We must do whatever is necessary to help them achieve their goal of having their kids recover. Do what your heart and your head tell you to do. You are stronger and wiser than you think! You can teach an old dog new tricks. Trevor has taught me plenty.

Kristine Lambert
(Mother of Team TMR's Oracle)

7

Mickey

Get Up You SOB, Because Mickey Loves You

Prologue

The setting is the mid-1980s, a time when corporate greed and self-ishness practically decimated my entire generation in the name of doing everything they could to produce as much corporate profit as possible. If this meant cutting costs, cutting salaries, outsourcing, cutting jobs, etc., so be it. The explanation was (and still is) that corporate management has one main task—to increase profits for the corporation's shareholders—no matter the fallout.

It was at this time that I lost my job and was unemployed for several months. One day I was taking a walk with my thirteen-year-old daughter, Nikki. She was crying over my plight and said to me, "Daddy, it isn't fair." I looked at her and said, "Nikki, you're right, it isn't fair, but it doesn't matter. What we have to do is learn from this and move forward. Let's allow ourselves two more days of crying, and then let's wipe away our tears, raise our fists, tell the world to stuff it, and do what we can do to move forward. Let's always remember that we should rely on ourselves first and make it happen. And furthermore, it's very important that we do it ethically, with compassion and concern for others." I didn't realize at the time the impression my words had made on Nikki.

The years that followed were not kind to us. Nikki worked hard, got into college, studied hard, and even worked as many as three part-time jobs at a time to get through. I tried to help her as much as possible, but with my situation, I was practically useless—all I could do was give emotional support, practical guidance, and whatever financial help I was able to provide. Nikki came through like a champ: she graduated college and became what I had hoped she would be— tough, ethical, and compassionate. Little did I know at the time that I was observing the development of a future WARRIOR mom.

The Story

I am a grandfather of four children, three boys and one girl. My youngest grandchild, Noah, has been diagnosed with ASD (Autism Spectrum Disorder). I live in the Bay Area in Northern California, which is 400 miles from Orange County, where my daughter, son-in-law, and grandson live. This distance, and the fact that I work full time, makes it impossible to be with them on a daily basis to assist with the required 24/7 effort it takes to help recover a child with ASD.

I feel that grandparents and other extended support persons are vital in the fight against autism. One of the issues we have as grandparents is that most of us are not able to deal with the recovery process 24/7. Some of you grandparents are able to, and do, in fact, do it. God bless you for what you are doing to help not only your grandchildren, but also your children.

Before I got the telephone call from my daughter telling me that Noah was diagnosed with autism, I had no idea what autism was. All I knew at the time was that Nikki was very distraught and in tears. As her parent, I became very emotional but hid my feelings because

Nikki was going through so much emotional stress and I didn't want to add to it by showing my own emotions. As a father, I wanted to help my daughter but was at a loss about what I could or should do. The only thing I could think of was to keep calm and be supportive. Inside, I was emotionally torn. For Nikki to be as emotionally distraught as she was, this ASD thing had to be terrible. Nikki was talking about losing her child to a black hole. She was distressed that all of the plans that she and Jason had for their child were going down the drain. Hearing this, I felt that stress on two counts: one, as a parent who was feeling the pain of his child losing a child, and two, as a grandparent who was affected by the pain and agony Noah was going through now and the uncertainty of his future. However, at the time, all I could do was listen—and be distraught.

What an eye-opener the following year was! First of all, at that time, which was about four years ago, the lack of general knowledge about autism and the common belief that autism was unrecoverable simply blew me away. Right from the start, Nikki and Jason jumped right in and gave everything they had in time, emotions, and money to fixing Noah. I felt terrible, as I didn't have either the time or the money to provide sufficient help. My wife and I talked with Nikki on the telephone daily, sometimes three or four times a day, and got a blow-by-blow description of what she was going through and the intense effort it required. It is incredible that she was able to do what she did.

While trying to help Noah, his parents kept getting archaic feedback from the mainstream medical community that there was nothing they could do and that they should stop wasting their time and money on a useless cause. This didn't fly with Nikki. It just pissed her off, and she adopted the attitude that if she and Jason were the only advocates for her son, then so be it. World, get out of our way, we're going to fix Noah!

What followed was amazing. Nikki dug into all the medical information she could find relating to autism. It wasn't long before

Nikki knew enough about autism that she could and did go nose to nose with medical doctors and other professionals, offering researched evidence when they were wrong in their beliefs. Hell, I'm not a technical slouch, but in my daily conversations with her, I couldn't understand half of what she was saying.

The worst part was the emotional roller coaster that my wife Ethel and I went through. The recovery process was not clean and consistent. The old adage—one step forward, two steps backward—was the norm. Every day was a different emotional experience. On Monday, we'd get a call and be told that Noah had progressed since going gluten-free. On Tuesday, we'd get a call that Noah had had a reversal. On Wednesday . . . etc., etc., etc. It was very difficult on us, because we wanted to offer words of comfort and support, yet Noah's parents were under so much stress that whatever we said would be bounced back with a resounding "Yeah, but . . . you don't understand what it's like. It's so complicated that whatever we do doesn't work most of the time."

What was particularly frustrating was that, as far as I could see, Noah was progressing over the long run. But the minor set-backs were a constant source of fear that he would revert and be lost forever. It was almost impossible to console my daughter when she was facing that experience. As a parent, I became very concerned about the stress my daughter was going through, and I feared that she would reach a point from which she wouldn't be able to recover. On the outside, I remained calm, but on the inside, I was panicking.

As I started to learn what autism is all about, I reflected, and it all made sense. Noah was a beautiful baby—I swear that he looked like a miniature replica of his dad—and made us all very happy. Everything seemed to progress normally, but during the end of his first year, he started exhibiting certain symptoms:

- He would cry all night and the only thing that seemed to calm him down was having a fan at the door of his room.

- He would throw items out of his play area, and when we put them back, he would throw them back out. We couldn't convince him to keep the items within his area. My thought at the time was that we had a very strong-willed child—little did I know.

- He would line up his toy cars and trains, and they had to be just so. If you tried to change anything, he would simply put them back the way he wanted them—no matter how many times you did it. I thought that he was going to be a research scientist—again, little did I know.

- When he got upset, it wasn't a normal temper tantrum—it was a complete meltdown, and there was nothing you could do to calm him down. Again, I thought he was a strong-willed child. Again, little did I know.

The tale goes on and on, as Noah showed all of the most common symptoms that children with ASD display. As I became more and more aware, I began to realize what we were dealing with, and I almost panicked, not for myself but for Nikki and Jason, for the life that might lie ahead for Noah, and also for all of those parents and children out there who were going through the same agony.

But Nikki did not give up. Instead, she started to challenge all the conventional wisdom that promoted the idea that there is no recovery from ASD. She found the autism support group Talk About Curing Autism (TACA), which anchored her. TACA showed her not only that there was light at the end of the tunnel, but also how to get there. The community provided emotional support because everyone involved in TACA had someone close to them who had ASD. They also offered stories of other parents who were dealing with ASD and examples of the progress and recoveries that were made. Finally, they provided Nikki with names of medical professionals who specialize in ASD so that she could get expert help from those who knew what the issues were and how to approach the problem.

This support gave her hope, because she now knew where to start and what to do to help Noah recover. I started to feel better, because now we began to see that there was light at the end of the tunnel, and although I realized that the road ahead was going to be one hell of a fight, at least it was a fight that could end in victory. I began to believe that we would win this battle, because I saw that Nikki was relentless in her pursuit to recover Noah. I also started to hear and read about other parents like Nikki, all of whom displayed the same strength, persistence, and "If you can't help me, then get the hell out of my way!" attitude. I don't know where they got their strength, but that strength was there, and that strength is the reason that their children started to recover.

I also learned, much to my dismay, that those dealing with autism are basically on their own, because the world out there is harboring all kinds of misunderstandings and lack of knowledge about autism and its causes and effects. It seemed that at every turn I would get all kinds of ridiculous responses to almost any issue I brought up about autism. The typical answer I got was, "Well, you can't prove what you just said." Now, my mother might have raised a fool, but she did not raise a complete idiot, and I do understand basic logic. No one seemed to want to accept that environmental issues, such as food, air, chemicals, and stress, could be factors in the development of autism. Now, I realize that some of these connections are not proven definitively and are still very controversial. However, I find it frustrating that people can't understand that the absence of definite proof doesn't mean the connection doesn't exist—it simply means that we don't yet know whether it does.

When the "professionals" can't give a parent the answer, doesn't the parent have to move forward and do the best they can do with what they have? These parents are put in the position of having to be research scientists, because their child's life is at stake and they can't get the answers they need anywhere else. Shouldn't they do the most logical thing instead of allowing the status quo to persist just because there is no definite proof? Many issues, ranging from vaccinations to food, air temperature, chemicals—the list goes on and on—are at play here. When parents change something in the environment and get positive results, what should they do? Ignore the results because there hasn't been a ten-year FDA-approved scientific research project? No, they should move forward, follow their gut, and do what seems to work, because no one else is giving them any answers.

What really frustrated me, and still does, are the almost violent rebuttals I got from people who seemed to be parroting the mainstream information without looking into the facts. I realized that most of these people simply didn't know what they were talking about and just blindly believed whatever they had heard from their friends and the media.

Noah's progress, meanwhile, has been phenomenal. Most people would no longer even notice some of the autism symptoms he still shows. He is a bright and very loving child. I'm amazed at how smart he is. One time, when he was about two or three years old, Noah asked me to help him with something on his iPad. I couldn't help him, so Noah showed me how to do it. (And I'm supposed to be the computer guru in the family—ha, ha!) We all got a laugh out of it and were very pleased at the way he was developing.

As I read more and more, I began to understand the world of parents who had children with ASD. These parents are just like Nikki and Jason—they are WARRIOR parents. These WARRIOR parents are becoming a growing and formidable army determined to win this war no matter what. Their stories are the same—desperation, lack of understanding and help from those professionals whom they grew up believing they could rely on to get information to solve their problems, and an inner strength that none of them knew they had. I encourage all of these WARRIOR parents to keep at it and keep sticking together in mutual support.

I also learned that these WARRIORS are seriously overextended and need lots of help in terms of extended support so that they can have more time and strength to help their children. I have come to believe that this is the role that grandparents, extended family, and friends should strive for. The most obvious way to help is to give emotional support by listening, but there are many other practical things that can be done:

- Offering financial support, if possible
- Learning the details of the child's diet and helping in the preparation of the food
- Shopping
- Babysitting, which requires that we learn about the physical issues, such as meltdowns, stimming, extreme diarrhea, poor muscle tone, poor balance, etc., and how to deal with them
- Participating in the autism support groups, which will promote a deeper understanding of what's involved in caring for a child with autism
- Learning about the therapy sessions
- Spending quality time with the children
- Learning and practicing the benefits of GF/CF/SF eating habits, which will promote not only better understanding, but also family unity, companionship, and health

Epilogue

The setting is now the year 2014. Noah is doing fantastic. Nikki has a better grip on the path required and the understanding of what it will take to continue. I have a good understanding of what autism is all about, and I am becoming very passionate about my role in the war to defeat it. I am normally a middle-of-the-road person, but not when it comes to autism. I am convinced that we can defeat it, and I'm also convinced that we are facing two formidable enemies: Greed and Lethargy.

Despite these challenges, Noah has made incredible progress, and my wife and I are overjoyed at how far he has come. Just yesterday, he was giving Nikki instructions on how to plan and prepare for this upcoming Halloween. When Noah was first diagnosed, we couldn't even get him to acknowledge us, and now he's telling us not only what to do, but also what to watch out for to make sure everything goes well. While it's true that he still has issues to overcome, the fact is that most people would not even realize that he has ASD if they just observed him in action.

Now, what about all the other children out there? What can we do about all this? As grandparents, we are in a subtly important role. We typically are not available 24/7 to help out, but we are also typically pillars of strength to look to for emotional guidance and support. Those grandparents who are already contributing by being involved 24/7 are doing an amazing job. In some cases, grandparents have even given up retirement so they can help their children and grandchildren.

To me, the basic problem is that the warrior moms and dads are on the front line and completely overwhelmed. They have to not only fix their kids, which is an intense effort by itself, but also do the research and argue with the doctors and the agencies that are supposed to be advocates for these children but often are another faction of resistance. My point is that the role of the warriors is to manage and fix their children. They don't have time to do the extended support things. They need help.

I compare this situation to an army going to war. The army doesn't simply give a bunch of weapons to the soldiers and say, "Go do it." It relies on an extended support staff to allow the front-line warriors fight the battle. As a thinking grandfather, I am that support person for my daughter and son-in-law, and it is my role to do whatever I can to give them relief and more time to be the front-line warriors.

We need to get organized and come up with strategies and tactics to stand any kind of chance. I absolutely believe that Team TMR is on the right track. You know the saying, "I'm up to my ass in alligators, and they're asking me to get out of the swamp!" Well, that's the position we're in with autism. At this time, everyone is a front-line soldier, and until the support mechanisms get there, it'll be a losing cause. The good news is that it can be done. Look at what Team TMR and the other autism support organizations are doing. They are providing practical front-line assistance, information and knowledge, money, and networking. We all have to start thinking the same way. In other words, we also have to start thinking about the strategic battle, which involves increasing public awareness, providing financial support, and offering the other kinds of support that the primary care providers need to maintain the strength and energy to continue the battle.

These goals are not limited to those of us directly involved. They also include the government mechanisms that must realistically understand the issues and provide the opportunities for our children to become healthy and productive citizens. Right now, one in forty-five of our children is diagnosed with ASD, and that number is getting worse and worse with each report. We have to fix this. There is no alternative option.

From what I can see, we do have the people who can do it. We must maintain the attitude that nothing will get in our way. WE WILL WIN THIS WAR!

Chuck Di Bari
(Father of Team TMR's Rocky)

8

"Yee Haw!"

Hope and Healing across Generations

MY OWN STORY ALSO STARTS WITH A BATTLE AGAINST A MYSTERIOUS, little-understood disease. When I became ill at eighteen months of age, it took the specialists three months to go from a diagnosis of the flu to virus X to finally polio. That was in 1950. My mother did the best she could, but there were four of us, living on a second-class navy man's pay. After the diagnosis, I spent the next six months in the hospital with paralysis in my right leg. The hospital stay was followed by years of physical therapy, surgeries, braces, and a fear of needles.

I wish my mom had told the doctors and nurses about my fears; I wish that someone had explained things to me or asked me why I was acting out as I grew older and more conscious of the difference in the length of my legs once the braces came off. But that's not how things worked in my family or in the medical field at that time. Back then, parents left their children in the hospital; there was no staying with the child. They kissed you goodbye, and if you were lucky, you saw them the next day. There was no Internet, so parents didn't have Google to help them connect with other parents facing the same things and get advice or support.

I traveled a long road of surgeries, pain, isolation, and loneliness. I would always have a limp and one leg that would never develop in size. Because of that, I grew up being no stranger to stares, nudges, or loud whispers I was meant to hear. I survived by retreating into my head to cope and block it all out—there I felt safe and didn't wear a brace, or limp, or have a skinny leg. I would later see and recognize that trait of withdrawing from the world in my great-nephew, Matthew, which helped create our special bond.

When my niece Terri had her son Matthew in 2003, she was a very different mother than my mother (her grandmother) was, and it was a very different time. From the moment the stick of the pregnancy test first turned blue, she was ecstatic. This would be her first baby. She was determined to do everything possible to bring a healthy baby into this world through an intervention-free natural childbirth. Books were read, doulas hired, and she was ready. Little did she know that motherhood's first curveball was headed her way. After twenty hours of Pitocin-filled labor, Matthew finally emerged via C-section. Terri's labor and delivery were polar opposites from what she had wanted, but that was only the tip of the iceberg.

The next part appeared after he received his vaccines. Matthew showed the first signs of damage after his four-month vaccinations, but it would take four years for him to receive an official diagnosis of autism and be on his way to recovery. At that time, the doctors would say that he had colic or that maybe he was lactose intolerant, but they couldn't explain why he was constantly screaming, why he did not sleep, or why he had trouble both nursing and tolerating the formula that they had to supplement with at times. My niece tried everything there was to try to settle him down: rocking, carrying him in a baby sling, running the vacuum to provide white noise. Nothing worked for long. It was hell. If things did get better, it was just about time for the next round of vaccines, and the cycle would start over again. It would be years before they would connect the dots between these behavioral shifts and vaccines.

At two, Matt, as he likes to be called these days, was still non-verbal and still in his own world most of the time. But he would be in the moment and respond to you if you were singing, so his mom incorporated music into mealtime routines.

Other adjustments were made as well. Since Matt still had trouble sleeping at night, his dad came up with the idea of bolting his dresser to the wall, removing anything potentially dangerous, and installing a high "Dutch door" in his room so they could have security in knowing Matthew would be safe if they did not hear him wake up in the middle of the night. That didn't happen often, however. When Matthew couldn't sleep, neither could Terri; I am not sure how she functioned during this time. Matthew slept for no more than four hours and never all at a single stretch.

A few new problems appeared around this time as well. Feeding became more difficult, because he would suddenly refuse or throw up foods that he used to enjoy in the past. He also was very restrictive in his eating, mostly requesting foods made from wheat and dairy. He had low muscle tone and extreme sensitivity. He reacted strongly to the feel of sand, grass, a former favorite blanket—it was almost as if touching them caused him pain. And yet he would scrape or cut himself and act as if he could not feel the pain at all!

Tantrums and aggression would become the norm. He would be fine one moment and then, out of the blue, start throwing anything he could find and knocking things over. It didn't matter what it was that was in his path. He was just that frustrated.

To help with his aggression, I'd take him out to the pool; we would sing "Hit the Road Jack" and smack the water as hard as we could to vent; the higher the splash, the louder we'd sing. We also used some other simple methods to help Matthew cope: his mom made him a blanket filled with poly beads for weighted compression on his body; his dad put a swing in his room so he could twirl around, as well as inflatable balls that he could kick without hurting himself or causing damage. We turned to music again and even came up with a special dance we'd do to Patsy Cline's "Walking after Midnight," complete with twirls and lifts in the air; I'd end it with a big "Yee Haw!" to signal we were done. We had an agreement that we'd only do the dance three times because he would not want to stop, so we started counting down. Three would become our magic number, because it gave him a definite limit for repeating tasks, twirls, or even the number of cookies he could have. He needed well-defined boundaries—it seemed to make him feel better to know what he could expect beforehand.

Another problem was the withdrawal. You could actually look in Matthew's eyes and see him withdraw, taking on a blank stare, shutting down, and retreating when he got overwhelmed. It was heartbreaking. There were times when the fog lifted from his eyes and he was "in the moment," such as, for instance, when he ran a fever. In those times, he became aware of you and would respond when you talked to him. Fevers were very rare, but when he did have them, they brought clarity.

Around this age he also started becoming obsessed with objects. First it was a bulb syringe, then it was a bottle of calamine lotion (after his second bout of chicken pox), then a toy phone, then a real lemon (the real lemon eventually had to be replaced by a fake one). And heaven help us if his object of the moment could not be found! Something about having them with him made him feel safe, secure, and comforted and gave him something tangible to hold on to. The obsessions would last for many years. We eventually found ways to use these items to increase Matthew's interactions with us: repeating the object's name or color, or playing "find," or figuring out who has the lemon or phone. We used the objects to do an activity first or to refocus his attention.

At three, Matthew was still nonverbal, but he showed comprehension. If you asked him to spin something purple or pick out a certain shape, he went right to it. To help reach Matthew, I started talking out loud, explaining everything we were doing step by step, counting, naming people in photos, pointing out if they had smiles or frowns on their faces, singing—anything verbal and repetitious. I was hoping he'd repeat the words and begin speaking. Matthew and I would go up and down the stairs and I'd count them out, one through thirteen. Months went by. Then one day, as we were going on up, I got to number ten and stopped, thinking, "This isn't working, I'm just talking to myself. I'm even tired of hearing me." Then I felt a tug on my hand, and Matthew said "eleven" and proceeded to count to the top. I cried, because the feeling of *I'm getting through* was fantastic.

Meanwhile, Terri was searching for answers, unwilling to settle or accept traditional medicine diagnosis or labels since they really offered no concrete help. She had been told that there was nothing to do and that autism was genetic. She would not accept that she could make no positive changes for her son. She was soaking up information like a sponge. Over the years, Terri had started to link certain things to certain behaviors and making adjustments. For instance, she changed their diet to eliminate foods containing red dye after she read about the dangers of this additive. She also got her son into speech and music therapies, as well as DIR/Floortime therapy. DIR/Floortime is an intervention technique focused on using play therapy to connect with the child. Parents and caregivers (rather than just therapists) take on key roles in the process. Matthew responded very well!

Finally Terri heard from another mom about a specialist, Dr. Kurt Woeller, who was six hours away in southern California. So off she went, picking me up along the way to keep Matthew occupied, since her initial visit would be three hours long, with only the first half of the appointment involving Matthew. I came along to help care for him so that she and the doctor could go over what Matthew would need, what foods had to be eliminated from their diets, and what tests would need to be performed.

For the next hour and a half, Matthew and I sang and danced to Patsy Cline, pitched pennies into the fountains of the medical building and made wishes, ate the special snacks his mom had packed—anything to keep him occupied and not screaming, as waiting was not easy for him back then. When his mom signaled to us that she was done, Matthew pulled off my straw hat, threw it up in the air, and yelled "Yee Haw!" because we were done. We all started laughing at that one, including Dr. Woeller and his office staff! After that visit, all of our lives began changing for the better.

Terri came out of that appointment feeling validated! For once, a doctor listened and did not act like she was crazy. He treated her like an equal and gave her many additional things to consider. She walked out with test kits that seemed to never end, but those test kits would help find out what was going on. She also had a plan for methyl B12 injections and an immune modulator called Low Dose Naltrexone (LDN) to deal with his auto-immunity issues. The tests confirmed what we had suspected—his immune system was attacking his own body. That was showing up as food allergies, as well as a very underactive immune response to viruses and the rarity of running fevers in response to common infections, including chicken pox (which he got twice)! But most importantly, Terri finally had *hope*. A fire had been lit, and she now had a direction to move in. She also had a lot more research to do.

That visit took place in the summer of 2008, when Matthew was almost five years old. The changes that were made had an immediate impact. When the new school year started, Terri had already implemented many of the therapies, and the preschool teachers took notice and asked what she had done. Prior to seeing Dr. Woeller, Matthew needed a special classroom; the sensory overload from simply walking by an integrated classroom made him scream. After starting biomedical treatments, Matthew easily transitioned from the autism classroom to an integrated one. His language skills exploded.

The family ran the tests, made adjustments, changed diet, added supplements, tried homeopathy and essential oils, and treated gut dysbiosis (microbial imbalance), which included very persistent yeast and clostridia. Many of those things led to improvements in language, sleep, attention, sensory issues, eating, behavior, etc. He was changing and developing in front of our eyes!

Of course, not every intervention meant improvement. There was a lot of trial and error. Everyone is unique, and their responses to various treatments vary as well. It was uncharted territory, much like my own battle with polio decades earlier. I could relate to Matthew in many, many ways. I could relate so much that Terri started looking at my own chronic health issues and seeing parallels. Based on her research and advice, I started taking some of the same supplements and changing my diet. My health conditions improved as well, making it much easier for me to keep up with Matthew or climb inside a tunnel to console hurt feelings.

Formerly skeptical family members also saw the changes in Matthew. They could not ignore the improvement they saw with their own eyes. Now they know better than to question Terri. In fact, they often e-mail or call when they need advice!

Today, at age eleven, Matthew plays two musical instruments and reads voraciously. He has developed social skills (he's a Boy Scout) and is a gentle, funny, and kind child. He is in a mainstream fifth-grade class and only receives occupational therapy in school as his last remaining therapeutic intervention. He's thriving! He is so loving to his family. We frequently get an "I love you" out of the blue, as well as lots of hugs and kisses. When he has had a bad day, he can tell us he needs time alone to "decompress" or asks for a hug. Those things alone are huge progress for a child who had once had a very hard time managing emotions. I'm not saying he never has meltdowns, but the difference is that now he recognizes the signs and knows what he needs to manage them. Matthew recently even had his first sleepover; granted, it was just with me, but it was still away from home—another milestone!

So that's what our journey together has been like so far. Frankly, had I not experienced it myself, I wouldn't have believed it. I now want to tell others to never give up hope. Matthew's journey is proof that recovery can happen. But in order for it to happen, the child needs an advocate in their corner, someone who will speak up for them if they can't; someone who learns, mostly by trial and error, what they need and when they need it; someone who will devote time every day to their routine needs and be able to balance a home, work, and family too. Recovery needs a Wonder Woman! That is what my niece is, and I am so proud of her. She has even turned this experience into a career, working in the autism world and helping others through her work, her blog, and her mentoring of other parents. She wants more families to know that a diagnosis of autism isn't the end—it is simply another beginning.

Looking back now, I find it amazing how far Matthew has come. A few months ago, he was having a hard day and said to me, "it's hard to be me." I told him, "I get it, Bud, it's still hard for me too, but we're going to get through it."

My message to those reading this book is to get involved. There's so much you can do, even if it's only giving mom and dad a break for a couple of hours. Their lives are filled to the brim, so the kids can use your help. Your family may not ask for help; you just have to jump in and offer it. Don't be afraid that you don't know everything. They will tell you what to do.

One final important thing. If they are doing a special diet, respect that. It is important for these kids and does make a difference, regardless of whether you believe in it or not. And yes, even "a little bit" will hurt.

The peace of mind that comes from knowing that someone capable and competent is taking care of their child so they can go shopping alone, take a nap, or just to have some time to sit in peace and quiet is worth its weight in gold. The pure love you receive back, the relationship you will develop, and the special things only you experience with your grandchild, niece, or nephew will stay in your heart forever. There is no feeling more special than connecting with a child who has a hard time connecting with those around them.

Kathryn Heck
(Aunt of Team TMR's Shawty)

9

Twilight
The Possible Dream

IT'S FALL IN THE UPPER PENINSULA OF MICHIGAN. THE WEATHER IS sunny, and there is a cool breeze. The Star Line ferry is about to leave St. Ignace for Mackinac Island. I am in my favorite seat, and I am, quite simply, in Heaven. This is one of my favorite places in the whole world. Not that I am a world traveler by any means. However, I have often had opportunities to go elsewhere, but my heart always brings me back to this beautiful, peaceful place. It is a trek that I make with my three sisters annually. We all share the same crazy love for this special place. I sit back to enjoy the cool breeze on my face for the twenty or so minute ride.

I absent-mindedly touch the silver bracelet on my left hand, thinking how odd it is to be by myself on this trip. I have a reason to be on my own, however, and it is a monumental one. I have a promise to keep.

It is always an exhilarating ride. The hydro-jets make it a fun crossing, and the sights of the beautiful mansions, the Grand Hotel, the boats, and the Round Island Lighthouse consume me. The Straits of Mackinac make you feel that you are in a place of powerful, extraordinary waters. At long last, I am there.

I walk up the pier and out onto the bicycle-lined street. You only hear the clip-clop of horse's hooves, not the roar of cars, on this amazing island. I am walking down the boardwalk heading toward the shore that faces the Mackinac Bridge. I love this walk to our sacred spot. A spot that holds so much promise and reverence for us. I can barely stand it now that I am so close. I am almost running now.

I reach my destination. My heart is racing. I have waited for so long, praying for this day. I look down at my bracelet. The words "Autism Awareness" are still there, as they have been since I put it on ten years ago. I take it off and rub it almost reverently, one last time. I close my eyes and say, "Thank you God, I am grateful." Getting close to the water, I throw my bracelet, my beloved symbol, into the air. It travels a ways before it falls into the water. I feel peace and a wonderful feeling of jubilation all at once. I say to the wind, "For Kale Zachary! For his recovery, for Kale, for all of them!"

I wake up. The bracelet is still on my arm. It was a dream. It most surely was, in that Kale is not fully recovered, not yet. He will be one day; it's just not this day.

Kale Zachary and his twin brother, Jaden Michael, were born on June 2, 2003. Becoming a grandparent, for me, was so wonderful. It was an exciting time. Their birth weight was good for twins. We were so relieved that they had made it to full term and were healthy. Life had a new rhythm to it. It was work, babies, family, and more babies. There wasn't always a lot of sleep, even for us grandparents.

They were thriving, and it was something to marvel at. The twins were such a joy—they were our first grandchildren, and I was taken back to the days of young motherhood with my own three. The twins' mom, Sadie, was born when I was twenty; her brothers by the time I was twenty-seven. My husband Les and I were so blessed.

What a sweet gift it was to be given back a part of your life that went by way too quickly; only this time the babies were little reminders of what their parents had been all those years ago. It couldn't have been any sweeter.

Our family was busy with the everyday logistics of having twins around. Sadie and Mikey were blessed to have such devoted helpers along with us grandparents. Time went by quickly, and those little boys were growing and changing. Their first birthday had come and gone. They were so cute. It was such a joy to walk in the door and hear their little feet come running so you could scoop them up and kiss their little cheeks. There were milestones and days filled with the sweetness of just simply being. All too soon, that changed.

The signs that something was wrong were subtle at first. Kale would not look at us when we called his name. We would tell him to go pick up his blanket, and, after we said it several times, his brother would just go get it for him. When I look back, I can see it play out in my mind. It is all so surreal. I would be so concerned one day, and on another day I would think I was overreacting. Sadie's instincts were already there, though we didn't always talk about the problems. I think it's like a survival mode you go into. Eventually, however, we started acknowledging how we were all feeling.

The hardest thing for me was Kale's lack of eye contact; it was hard because he did have it before. He also started doing what we learned later was stimming—repetitive movements or vocal tics. And he kept lining up his Matchbox cars and Little People toys in long rows or in circles around him.

Sadie and Mikey began searching the Internet. Sadie filled out questionnaires that gave you a number score for how many symptoms your child had. She was worried. At the time, Sadie was a manager at a popular restaurant in town. Her degree was in business administration, not special education. However, she was discovering many things that would later on become second nature. I worked in special education, but I didn't know much about Kale's symptoms.

It really was a time of trying to get information, struggling to digest it, and praying that it wouldn't turn out to be true. One day my sister stopped by. Her degree was also in special education. I had Kale sitting on the counter and was talking to him, trying to engage him. I turned and looked at her. I saw it in her eyes. She was very concerned. We all were.

Shortly after that, my niece Beth, a speech and language pathologist, came over to see Kale. She was trained to work with the little ones. My daughter called me that very day. Beth had explained to her that the "A" word was overused, but admitted that Kale had delays for sure; they discussed many things that day.

Sadie and I talked for a while. She was stoic, close to acknowledgement. I couldn't even breathe when I hung up the phone. I wanted to scream, "Why Kale? Why them? Why us?" It was the first time, but not the last, that I would ask those questions. A few months later, Kale Zachary was diagnosed with autism by a very capable, caring team at LaRabida Children's Hospital in Chicago, Illinois. The diagnosis came as no surprise. The question was not so much whether Kale had autism, but whether he would ever be able to talk.

On the drive home from the consultation, the boys were happy. We realized that life would be different from now on, but it was going to be all right. It was going to take all of our strength, however, especially Mikey and Sadie's. As Kale's grandmother, I looked into that little face with the beautiful brown eyes, and I swore that I would be there for him. The trick was going to be balancing autism with the rest of life. How would we support Kale, and Sadie, and Mikey and have enough time and energy for ourselves and our other children? We would find that balance and push forward every day.

Time went on. The boys turned three. It was around that time that Kale was diagnosed with apraxia (which affects the child's ability to speak, to get the sounds out). That diagnosis was hard to hear, but once again we had to put our fears aside for the time being and just get on with life. If we didn't, all we would do was worry. Instead, we reached out for help. Sadie and Mikey went to their first AutismOne conference in 2006, and it helped them in so many ways. They brought me back a gift: it was the "Autism Awareness" bracelet that would later show up in my dream. I loved it. The bangle style was perfect for me. I put it on that day and have worn it every day since.

Over time, we started asking questions. What do we do? How can we, Kale's grandparents, help? There is no instruction manual on how to be an autism family; you just become one. How do you help your loved ones when you yourself feel so low? Make no mistake about it, the whole family was affected, as well as caring friends. It was a huge adjustment for everyone, especially for Sadie and Mikey, but it was their baby, and they had to fight for his recovery. They began the quest, and we would help them by providing what was needed by loving and supporting all of them as best we could. Even though we were afraid, there was also real hope in our hearts. Hope was the foundation upon which we would build the fight for Kale's recovery.

Of course, it wasn't as though I sat down and mapped out my course, my strategy. It didn't work that way. We all just jumped in with both feet. Each day brought some news to adjust to, some small accomplishment or setback. We faced the challenges together. My husband has always been a huge support for all of us. He learned early on to care for the twins, never backing away from what Kale needed. The boys were lucky: they had not only us, but also another set of loving grandparents. There were also aunts, uncles, cousins, and friends to lean on. From the very beginning, Sadie and I had a habit of checking in with each other. She would call or text me before she went to sleep. Then I would usually hear from her sometime in the morning. Usually we just checked in about the day and what was going on, but it worked as a great support for both of us.

One of the first practical steps we took was Early Intervention. The professionals who became involved with the boys—Jaden had some problems with speech too—were very helpful. Jaden responded very quickly to speech therapy, and that was a relief.

In those days, I was quickly learning all kinds of new things. My mind worked hard to keep up with all the new concepts. Sadie was off and running, literally. She was working but spent as much time as she could with the boys, and the rest of the time researching. She would hunt down websites that had anything that could be helpful. For my part, often the best thing I could do was to be there and listen, as well as to just love Kale and Jaden. That was also the easiest thing that I had to do—love those boys.

I helped out in other ways too. Friday night was my night to be with them while Sadie and Mikey were working. I would often stay into the morning hours. I would get Jaden settled, but often Kale would not cooperate, so he'd wake Jaden back up. Then I'd rock them both to sleep. Often they would play with my autism bracelet. I was a younger grandma, but it was still hard to keep up. We didn't know it then, but sleep, or the lack of it, was going to be one of the biggest struggles that Kale would face.

We learned basic sign language to help Kale communicate. He did very well with it. Sometimes I took Kale to speech therapy. On the way home, he would start fussing as we went by a restaurant. He wanted fries, but couldn't tell me using his words. You just had to know what he wanted.

It was not always easy to get Kale to therapy, however. Some of his therapies were in their home, but not always. Logistics were a challenge sometimes, especially with Mikey working nights. Every mom and grandma knows that the nights can be the hardest. They did not live with us, but Les and I were there a lot, and sometimes we would take the boys overnight so their parents could do something or just sleep!

Despite these difficulties, I enjoyed my time with the twins very much. Sometimes it would be such fun when a couple of their aunts and uncles, cousins, and/or grandparents were there together watching the boys. There was love all around, and we all have special memories. Keeping up with my own family responsibilities and connections with friends was always important to me, although difficult at times. At the time, I was also working at a school full time, helping students who needed me throughout the day.

When they were three, the boys were enrolled in an early childhood program through their school district. It was a very hopeful time. Jaden's communication skills had improved a lot by this point. He was getting extra support, and it showed. He was progressing as hoped. Kale went into the class that best suited his needs at the time and had a very supportive team.

Soon Sadie and Mikey began looking into alternative recovery methods. It would put them on a whole new journey. Biomedical was the first big protocol. I have to admit, I didn't always understand what was going on. Sadie would tell me about something interesting she found and why it was important. Next thing I knew, my head would be spinning, but I would catch on. It wasn't always easy. There were changes in their family as well. Sadie was working toward her master's degree in Special Education, and Mikey got a new job. It helped them so much to have good health insurance, since it had been a struggle to pay for therapy and supports for Kale. Sadie has since become a developmental therapist and autism advocate, helping other little ones and their families.

In the meantime, Kale learned to communicate with some words. It was such a joy every time he used a new one. We were finally able to understand what he was saying or trying to say. A lot of other new things were coming up: diet changes, sign language, supplements, communication devices, practitioners, swimming lessons, horseback riding therapy, adaptive swings—and that's just the tip of the iceberg.

There were also nutritionists, because Kale had sensory issues and wouldn't eat many foods. That was to become one of Sadie's biggest passions and hardest challenges—the things that went into her children's bodies. "Gluten-free" and "casein-free" weren't just words; they became a way of life. There were a lot of doctor's appointments as well. Kale quickly learned that the doctor's office was not somewhere he wanted to be. It would take two people to get him through the visits. They had to papoose him to draw blood: they laid him on a flat board that had thick Lycra bands that wrapped around his body and used Velcro to fasten him tightly. He could not move his body while in the papoose, and only one arm was free. It was a traumatic experience for all of us.

As Kale got older, IEP (Individualized Education Plan) meetings became a part of each school year. Correct placement and proper support at school for children with autism is always trial and error. Kale was blessed with many caring educators, many of whom loved him like their own. But there is always so much to do and consider for a child with disabilities, so not every situation was great, and it took diligence to get him in the right setting. Having teachers with extensive professional development and experience supporting students with autism is both necessary and vital to their success. Modifying the physical environment within the classroom, providing the right academic supports, arranging sensory movement breaks throughout their day, providing transition supports when moving throughout the building, and putting together social skills groups are all things that needed to be discussed within the IEP meetings to make sure Kale had the right amount of support to become a successful learner in the academic setting.

A huge discovery for Kale's parents was homeopathy. Homeopathic practitioners are enlightened in regards to children with disabilities. I think they are valuable for many reasons, the most important of which, to me, was the treatment of Kale's whole being rather than individual symptoms. Mikey and Sadie related to this line of therapy like nothing they had tried before. The confirmation that Kale's body could heal from anything that had harmed his system was so important to them, because there was a lot of damage that had to be reversed. Even an antibiotic could harm his system. Things went into his body, but didn't come back out—we would later learn he had trouble with his detox pathways. Sadie and Mikey addressed this and Kale soared into a healthier being.

These alternative ways of healing took into account his whole medical history and the way he reacted to everything. I still laugh as I think of the words we used when we first heard of homotoxicology. Les called it "voodoo." Sometimes the label fit, but more often than not Kale would benefit from these treatments. I can say that adjusting to new things gradually became easier for us. We kept up fairly well. Of course, not all new discoveries worked for Kale; there were a couple that didn't. As with so many things in life, we would cry, rail at the hardship, and then pick back up where we left off. It is so much better to see the glass as half full rather than half empty. After all, Kale is making huge strides every day. He continues to amaze everyone around him. Every victory for Kale is a victory for all of us, and we feel them deeply. We also make sure not to let autism define who Kale is or how life will be for him.

Of course, there are still challenges. For instance, holidays and family gatherings can be hard for him to handle due to anxiety, sensory overstimulation, dietary restrictions, and lack of sleep, but even these have gotten much easier for Kale. We have many wonderful times with him. He especially likes coming to our house for sleepovers with his cousins.

Kale is twelve years old now. There have been many layers of triumph, despair, joy, disappointment, and happiness. It is often the little victories that mean the most. Kale has them often. It is important to remember that through it all, Kale will have experienced hardship, but also great joy and happiness, and that his life is uniquely his.

There is one thing I can say for certain: homeschooling has been an amazing decision for him. The decision to homeschool Kale was made last year when he started puberty and his anxiety escalated. He loves homeschooling and is very successful at it—the accomplishments just continue. Sadie has nurtured his love of art, and he completes the most beautiful paintings daily. I get to help her homeschool Kale one day a week, and the days that I spend with him are very special. When he comes home from school, Jaden always wants to see what his brother has done during his school time. If Kale is not finished with school at that time, Jaden sits down and helps him finish his work. They enjoy that time together.

To all families who are just starting a similar journey, I would say, don't lose heart or hope. Just focus on one day at a time. Hold onto each other and reach out to others when you feel you can't go on anymore. Family and friends will pick you up and support you until you can stand alone again. It is hard to let people in, for if you do, you show them the depth of your pain. That is very difficult, but it is worth it. Sadie has the love and support of her brothers and sisters, aunts and uncles, cousins, and Grandpa. Additionally, Sadie has found support in TMR moms. She also has a group of local autism moms, called "The Illinois Autism Mamas," that she leans on for guidance. She and Mikey also have their parents, friends, and wonderful neighbors. I try to be there for my daughter, and she is always there for me. It brings us peace.

We recently got our family together. It is always such a sweet time to have all of our kids and their families come together. During the gathering, Kale was riding in our golf cart with Papa and his cousins. They were going along, and he decided to throw all his Pokémon cards in the air, laughing. Papa stopped, and the kids piled out to help Kale pick them all up. That's how it goes when Kale is surrounded by people that love him. They support him in any way he needs. There are many times like this when Kale is just one of the kids. These are special moments.

As grandparents, we can only hope that we have given our children and grandchildren, in some small measure, whatever they need. I know one thing for sure—they will always have our unconditional love and support.

This year, I feel, will be a big one for Kale Zachary. He is doing all kinds of amazing things. His spontaneous speech exploded this past summer. In years past, his verbal communication has been limited to imitation of sounds and words, as well as to his communication device (due to his apraxia). He finally started talking in the month of June, when he turned twelve years old. He has been working with an amazing Speech Pathologist/Audiologist for a little over a year, and everything has finally come together after years of hard work. He has begun requesting what he wants and needs spontaneously with one-word phrases and some two-word phrases. He now has over seventy spontaneous words on the word list Sadie has been tracking for him. Hearing his voice is one of the most beautiful sounds for all of us.

I know that Kale will continue to grow into his own person; he just takes a little bit longer than others to conquer some of the developmental milestones. Strides will be taken and goals will be met. I'm sure of it.

Through it all, I have worn my bracelet. It is my symbol of hope, reminding me of the possibility of Kale's recovery from autism. I believe that I will get the chance to live out my dream someday. I will take the bracelet to my island and throw it to the wind. Kale's journey is still ongoing. His recovery will keep progressing, and his life will be full. He will guide us to what he needs to live a fulfilling life. I rejoice for now in the simple joy of loving him and being his Grama (our family spelling).

Judy A. Smith
(Mother of Team TMR's Guardian)

10

Crackle and Pop
"No Mom and Dad— Just Grammy and Papa"

THE NURSERY WAS ALL SET FOR THE ARRIVAL OF OUR DAUGHTER AND son-in-law's firstborn. We were all so excited. Our daughter lived an hour and a half away, so the week before her due date, Crackle went to stay with her and her husband. She was not going to take a chance and miss the birth of this baby. He was born exactly one week late. Alexander was finally here, with his big blue eyes and lots of curly brown hair, so precious. It was instant love.

I (Crackle) stayed with our daughter and son-in-law over the next several months. I wanted to spend every moment with my grandson and help my daughter. Pop would come visit us every weekend. We had so many fun outings together, like going to Sesame Street Live. It was always sad when Pop had to leave Sunday night.

Alexander was a very active baby. I remember how he would crawl up to me requesting his bottle ("babas," as he would call it), playing peek-a-boo and patty-cake, and looking for his toys. He really liked playing a game where we would throw the ball up the stairs and laugh watching it bounce back down. Alexander also loved to play in the cupboards, banging the pots and pans. In short, he did the things that all babies do.

When Alexander woke up for his nightly feedings, I would go into his room and sit with my daughter. I truly did not want to miss one moment of this time, because I realize that time goes by so fast. One night, Alexander kept waking up. As my daughter, son-in-law, and I were all sitting in Alexander's room at 3:00 a.m., I looked at both of them and said, "Yep, your life is not going to change." It was a joke between the three of us, because they kept telling me, "When we have our son, he is going to have to adjust to our life. How hard can it be to have one baby?" However, here we were, sitting there, the three of us, exhausted. I told them, "Welcome to parenthood."

Alexander started walking at around nine months. As soon as he could walk, he became fascinated by soccer. He would kick and dribble the ball around with his little feet, and we were sure he was going to be a soccer pro. We spent hours playing in the yard.

At this time, Alexander was hitting all his milestones, except for speech, where he was definitely delayed. I went to most of his doctor's appointments with my daughter. I listened as she questioned the doctor about the speech delay. The doctor kept telling her, "You have a healthy, happy baby." He is a boy, the doctor said, and boys start talking later than girls. My daughter also wondered why her son was having so many ear infections, and again the doctor's response was that it was normal. Then the questions about vaccines came up. I remember my daughter in tears, telling the doctor, "I don't feel comfortable giving him four vaccines at every appointment. It just feels like too many." The doctor replied, "Don't worry, this is normal, and we do it all the time." My daughter asked her for more information, and the doctor gave her a piece of yellow paper that failed to provide any.

Nine hours after this particular visit, Alexander broke out in a rash over his entire body. We took him to the hospital, but the doctors said it might be eczema and sent him home. We now believe the rash was a reaction to the vaccines.

We were all stunned when Alexander was given the official diagnosis of autism at the age of two and a half. Tears, tears, and more tears. It seemed like a nightmare, and then reality set in, and we thought about what we could do to fix, heal, or reverse the problem. As grandparents, we have always been able to fix every problem or at least put a Band-Aid on it. The hurt we felt as we saw our daughter in pain and struggling, along with the hurt of what had happened to our grandson, was devastating. It was heartbreaking. Why did this happen? It was not supposed to happen.

After a couple of days of breakdowns, our daughter found her strength and began to act. She researched and then scheduled doctors' appointments and therapies; she and our son-in-law attended many autism conferences. She researched different diets and supplements, and read all the information pertaining to autism that she could get her hands on. I think going to Temple Grandin's seminar gave her hope.

As time went on, Alexander started to show improvement. Most of the therapies, like speech therapy, occupational therapy, and Floortime, seemed logical and beneficial. Other things we tried, such as eating therapy, were not so successful. And some others we just rolled our eyes at.

One of the things we tried was the supplements, which were a nightmare at first. Sometimes we took Alexander up north for the week or weekend. Our daughter gave us a list with specific directions about the supplements he needed to take; it seemed to include about fifteen to twenty things a day. The number was—and sometimes still is—mind-boggling. We had to give digestive enzymes at every meal, for instance, as well as Gaba and L-Theanine at night to calm Alexander and help him sleep. On top of the supplements, there was also a specific diet to follow. There was always a favorite treat or food that he could no longer have. This was heartbreaking, especially when he begged us for some of his favorite foods: pizza, Goldfish, or Cheez-Its.

We did not mean to disrespect our daughter's wishes, but sometimes we caved in when it came to the diet. Here are a few of the things we got caught doing. While his parents were on vacation, I put Cheez-Its in his school lunchbox for a little surprise. When we picked him up from school that day, the teacher told me that Alexander had the biggest smile on his face when he opened his lunch. The following week, when our daughter went to pick Alexander up from school, that teacher told her how happy he was to have Cheez-Its in his lunch. Later, we got the phone call from our daughter, and she was not happy with us. Another time, when we were watching Alexander while our daughter was attending the AutismOne conference in Chicago, we were driving and discussing what special treat we should get Alexander for the weekend. We were trying to decide between pizza and Cheez-Its.

We did not realize that Alexander was in the backseat making a video of our conversation. Even worse, he made a video of himself eating pizza at our kitchen table. In trouble again. Now we check the iPad before he leaves our house.

As parents, we have always supported our daughter and son-in-law with whatever they need for Alexander, whether it is picking him up from school or taking him on the weekend to give mom and dad a well-deserved break. We see how they struggle with autism every day. We know how difficult it can be. The supplements and the diet alone are so time consuming.

We have also traveled to many doctor's appointments with our daughter and her husband. We sometimes get to listen to what the doctors say, and we understand the treatments (not entirely, but we try). Most of the time, we watch our grandson so our daughter and son-in-law can talk with the doctor. I remember that, years ago, there were many times when I had to help my daughter hold my grandson down while he was kicking and screaming during blood draws. This is not easy, and it is a side of autism most people don't see.

Despite the difficulties we have had to face, our grandson has brought so much joy and laughter into our lives. We love watching the videos he makes. He has a bunch of stuffed animals that he names and films, changing his voice to mimic the way he thinks they would sound. One of our favorite videos that he made had him doing yoga, with deep breathing included. It was a thirty-minute video, and we were amazed at how well he did.

We also have a lot of fun together. Some of his doctor's appointments have taken us on long family trips to places like Chicago and New York. We were amazed when Alexander walked all over New York City without complaining. It was his mom who caused some trouble. She was apprehended by security at the Statue of Liberty for having a knife in the backpack (it was there for cutting up the apples she brought as a snack for Alexander).

This past summer, when we took Alexander to our cottage, one of his favorite places to visit, Pop brought along an Elvis CD. Alexander loved listening to song number eight, "Suspicious Minds." He played it over and over all summer. Just before he was to return to school in the fall, we had a family get-together at the home of our daughter's friend. They have a recording studio in their home. We were all taking turns singing karaoke. Finally, someone put on "Suspicious Minds," and Alexander got up, grabbed the microphone, and sang the whole song. We all had tears of joy. He then proceeded to take a turn on the drums.

It's important to remember that these kids are in there, even when they may seem unaware of their surroundings. In reality, they are very aware, and in time positive and new things will come out.

Alexander is now thirteen, and his parents have found a great school for him in Naples, Florida. They are now building a home there, so his dad is commuting back and forth from Michigan. As for Crackle and Pop, we sure miss our daughter and Alexander and are contemplating moving to Florida in the near future. We plan on spending a lot of time there this winter.

To all of you grandparents out there (we know that some may have it worse than others), just try to do the best you can for these children. They need us so much. We have had those bad days with the humming, and the tantrums, and all the other similar behaviors that autism brings. We love our daughter, son-in-law, and grandson. We would still be there for them doing most of these things if autism were not in our lives. We hope for a day when our grandson is healthy and autism is no longer in our lives. But it is today, and we will continue to support and be there for them. This is the role that every grandparent should play. We are so proud of the Thinking Moms' Revolution. We are not alone anymore.

Fred and Mary Kay Ciaramitaro
(Parents of Team TMR's Snap)

11

Pete

Helping My Daughter's Family Walk on Water

AFTER THE MIRACLE OF THE LOAVES AND FISHES, JESUS WAS TIRED. HE wanted to go up on the mountain to relax and pray. He told His disciples to get into the boat and that He would catch up with them later. They cast off and were on their way. When the disciples saw the figure of Jesus strolling on top of the water and coming toward them, they thought it was a ghost. When they recognized Him, Peter asked the Lord's permission to join Him, and when he got the OK, he stepped out of the boat and began tiptoeing across the water toward his Master. Suddenly, the wind began to blow, and the waves picked up. Peter panicked, began to drown, and cried, "Lord save me!" Jesus reached out His hand, picked him up, and said, "Oh, you of little faith, why did you doubt me?" Faith, trust, and confidence come before anything else.

Peter is my kind of guy. In the Bible, he always seems to insert his foot into his mouth at every important crossroad. If you are familiar with the Bible, you know what I mean. He was *human*. Yet the Lord loved him so much that He built His Church on Peter's belief in Him and the virtues of faith, hope, and love.

Hope is the mantra of the Thinking Moms . . . as it should be. Hope begins with what these moms have witnessed firsthand: miracles do happen! You must believe your loved ones suffering with iatrogenic autism are being helped by the love, care, and prayers that you have provided for them. You must believe that all the prayers of all the parents are being heard! In my experience, the Thinking Moms seem to be inviting all religions to join in this quest to support their children. This makes perfect sense. What else can unite the world if not a mother's plea for help and understanding for her sick child? This plea is universal, pure, and incorruptible.

My name is Don Joyce (eighty-four) and my wife's name is Sue (seventy-five). We are the parents of Lisa Joyce Goes (the Rev) and in-laws to her terrific husband, Dave. We retired in 1989 and built our dream home in a community called Sugar Springs, Michigan. It had twenty-seven holes of golf, an Olympic-sized swimming pool, a restaurant, and other delightful retirement amenities. It was quiet and peaceful, and we expected to spend our final years there. God, it seems, had a different plan in mind.

It must have been in the 1990s that I heard the word "autism" for the first time. It was probably a newscast presented with little fanfare about a sad disease affecting a few children. It left no lasting impression on me. In 2006, my grandson Noah was born. There were no complications, and he was considered a normal child. When he was one year old, his well visit resulted in profound physical illness. He got a fever, his eyes rolled back into his head, there was swelling at the injection site, and he experienced uncharacteristic lethargy for seventy-two hours. He did not make a sound during those seventy-two hours! Then he began screaming, nonstop.

At the age of two, a life filled with illness seemed to be Noah's destiny. The pain in his belly never subsided. His parents took him to doctor after doctor, specialist after specialist. While they tried to have hope, it was clear the exhaustion of caring for Noah and his extraordinary behavior and medical needs was taking a toll on them. Noah's sister and brother had no idea what was happening to their family, but they knew it wasn't good.

To make matters worse, visits to the pediatrician only exacerbated the problem. It took Lisa a long time to understand the genesis of his illness. During our trips to visit the doctors, we could see that she was fully engrossed in learning all she could about the true epigenetic roots of autism and understanding how her completely healthy child had been victimized by a system of pharmaceutical companies, government agencies, and the medical industry. All of them were working in concert to address the "autism issue" with no compassion or concern.

As parents, we were concerned about the exhaustion and stress that were taking a toll on Lisa. Dave shares these concerns, but a man's major role is to provide the funds necessary to support his family and pay the thousands of dollars necessary for Noah's treatments. He is doing that every single day, while Lisa continues to look for answers and support. They work together, but they have to be apart to make it happen, though they always come together to laugh, and talk, and enjoy one another's company.

In 2012, Lisa and her mother had a conversation. Lisa asked whether we would be willing to live with them and give them the support they needed, based on our capabilities. Dave would finish off their walkout basement, converting it into an apartment. We considered all of the ramifications and decided to put our house up for sale in September of 2013. We sold the house in October 2013, along with everything else that would not fit into our new digs.

We moved in November, and the fun began. It was as if we were starting a whole new family. While helping Lisa and Dave with the ongoing medical and behavioral issues autism presents, we also learned about the impact that Noah's illness had on his siblings, which is monumental. There are no social events that we can participate in as a family. None.

Unfortunately, the social isolation comes along with the territory. Most people just don't know how to interact with a child with autism. They would be overwhelmed by the dietary restrictions, special needs accommodations, and the constant vigilance over where he is and what he is doing.

Grandparents can play an important role just by being there, even though they do not have the speed to catch up with a kid who runs 100 miles a day. No kid is faster or stays awake longer than Noah (Lisa tells me this is due to his mitochondrial problem and his metabolic processing difficulty). But grandparents can do lots of other things that can help take the load off of the parents. For instance, my wife and I take Noah's brother and sister to karate practice. When my wife is feeling up to it, she folds the laundry. While my daughter takes Noah to his many therapy and medical appointments, we watch the kids.

If you are wondering what you can do, just show up and ask, "How can I help?" Then be prepared to do whatever they need. Don't take it personally when they are cranky. No one can truly understand the immense pressure these families endure day in and day out.

I have been intrigued over the past few years by the absence of a satisfying definition for the word "autism." After reading several books on the subject, I still could not come up with an answer to what it really means. So I asked my daughter, who is a walking encyclopedia of autism. She told me that autism is a word that describes behaviors that are caused by a combination of iatrogenic and epigenetic factors. Huh? That sent me directly to the dictionary.

"Genetic" refers to the inherited makeup that is passed down to each human being from their ancestors. Genes are constant from one generation to another and essentially remain the same. Genetics do not cause regressive autism, but genes are subject to invasion when attacked by environmental changes, viruses, bacteria, or a new toxin, which can alter the physical structure of DNA. These changes are then passed on to future generations. This is epigenetics, which literally means "above" or "on top of" genetics.

"Iatrogenic" refers to a medical disorder caused by a physician's treatment. In the case of autism, the "iatro" is a (preventive) medical attack, such as a vaccine, which can have disastrous effects on those kids who are sensitive to the viruses and toxins contained in the vaccines. What results is severe damage to their immune system, gastrointestinal tract, central nervous system, and neurological function.

Autism is preventable, treatable, and curable, according to my daughter.

All that said, the future is unknown, so there is no sense in worrying about it. Living in the present moment with faith, hope, and above all, love—no matter what tomorrow brings—this is what gets us through. If you are able to do so, I ask all grandparents to be there for your children when they need you. All we can do is to keep on HOPING! And don't be afraid to walk on water when you need to.

Don Joyce
(Father of Team TMR's Rev)

12

Roxie

Blessed

"For I know the plans I have for you," declares the Lord, "plans to prosper you and not to harm you, plans to give you hope and a future."

—Jeremiah 29:11

SO MANY PEOPLE USE THE EXPRESSION "WE ARE BLESSED" THAT IT HAS become a cliché. For us, however, it is truth carved in stone. We have so much for which we are grateful. First and foremost, we have each other, and then our family, who are all healthy and thriving. We have a wonderful son, daughter, daughter-in-law, son-in-law, and five grandchildren. We are fortunate that they all live close to our home, so there is no scheduling of out-of-town trips to see them.

We have also faced some struggles, however. Sometimes you think that your life's journey is proceeding at a nice pace, and then all of a sudden your world falls apart. As if it were yesterday, we remember 9/11. We remember it, however, for another reason besides the catastrophe that rocked our country. We were on our way to our daughter Heidi's home to babysit our grandsons while she ran a few errands. We were looking forward to spending time with Carson, who was two years old, and the newest member of our family, nine-month-old Gannon. Listening to the radio, we heard the broadcaster announce that the World Trade Center towers were hit by low-flying planes. As soon as we arrived at Heidi's, we turned on the television and to our horror realized that in one dreadful moment the world had altered significantly for these two little boys. What we did not know was that Gannon's world was about to change in yet another significant way.

Gannon was a loving and beautiful baby—big blue eyes, curly hair, and a smile that would light up the room. He was fun and funny. With much pride, we watched him develop during those early months into a spirited little guy. But then something started to seem amiss. When Gannon was around fifteen months old, he began to change, and he continued to regress throughout the next several years. Our cute little man was ignoring us. He was irritable, absent, and obsessed with lining up his toys. He didn't talk, he didn't make eye contact, and he didn't laugh, smile, or engage. Instead, he screamed and screamed. He screamed a lot! Sometimes he ran around the house flapping his arms as though a big bad wolf were chasing him. He was scared, and so were we. What in the world was happening? Reluctant to say anything to his parents, we wondered to ourselves if he might be deaf. When we called him, he did not even flinch. When his little face grimaced with tension, we wondered if he was in pain. We were worried.

Finally, we felt compelled to say something to Heidi and Doug. We asked if they had had Gannon's doctor check his hearing. They were way ahead of us, as we knew they would be, and they had already been having Gannon checked by his pediatrician. We were all perplexed.

We learned from Heidi that when he was fifteen months old, Gannon was given five vaccines. Soon after, his parents noticed that he was losing eye contact and (something we didn't know) no longer had solid stools. At the age of three, he was evaluated at school, and his parents were told that he was speech and language impaired. Plus, he had to get through each day with constant diarrhea.

Heidi and Doug suffered along with their son. Heidi was a true warrior! She was the CIA, FBI, county sheriff, and a PI all wrapped into one determined mother. She also prayed a lot.

For years, we observed all the modifications the family was making, from changing their diets (Gannon had a severe gluten intolerance) to the numerous protocols they were undertaking at the recommendation of different doctors. The many changes they incorporated into their lives were the direct result of a phone call Heidi received from one of Gannon's teachers saying that she believed Gannon might be autistic.

This phone call was followed by what Heidi says was the worst day of her life. She was home doing laundry when the phone rang. A lady on the other end of the line said, "I have your son. I found him walking on Benstein Road." Benstein Road is a main road about three long blocks from their house. Needless to say, we cannot imagine the anxiety Heidi must have felt. When she arrived to pick up Gannon, she was greeted by two police officers. She was sure they would judge her as being a horrible mother. Without saying a word, however, they handed Gannon back to her and allowed the two of them to return home. Gannon was safe, but life was surely about to become more complex!

This episode was a glimpse into what was to come. Gannon struggled with a variety of issues. He was a "runner": his parents could not take him to a store without him immediately bolting off in another direction. He was restless and could not sit still in a movie theater or at church. It also took a very long time to settle him down and get him to fall asleep at night. On one occasion, he moved a chair to the back door so he could step up high enough to push the garage door button and escape. His parents found him at a neighbor's house. The neighbors had brought him into their home and called the police—they didn't recognize Gannon standing in the dark on their backyard deck dressed only in pajamas.

His parents knew he needed help. Soon, Gannon was visiting doctor after doctor, going through chelation therapy and hyperbaric oxygen therapy (HBOT), taking a number of different supplements, and eating a completely modified diet.

Despite the difficulty of all these adjustments, and despite Gannon's diagnosis of Pervasive Developmental Disorder (PDD), he has been a gem of a grandson. A real character! We have so many funny Gannon stories that we could write a book about his antics.

Yes, he gets in trouble, just like any other kid. One day when the family came over to our house for a visit—we think Gannon was around seven at the time—he got into the toothpaste in our upstairs bathroom and proceeded to channel Picasso, painting in toothpaste all over the mirror, one wall, and the sink. Beautiful designs, we might add. No one noticed, and the family left. In a few minutes our phone rang. It was Heidi wondering if we had been upstairs in the bathroom. She said they were on their way back to our house so Gannon could clean up the mess he had made. Gannon confessed in the car on the way home. In they walked. Gannon, not saying a word, proceeded to go upstairs. He did a nice job of cleaning up. In my best Grandma voice, I said, "Gannon, you may have made a mess, but you owned up to it and you cleaned it up, and that's a good thing." He looked at me and, as serious as a judge, said, "I'm going to jail!" Then he walked down the stairs and out of the door. We could not help but laugh after the family left the house for the second time that day.

Gannon has other talents as well. He is very good on the computer and has been using one since the age of three. Honest! During another visit, he sat down at our computer and changed an icon that read "Patti" to one that read "Patti/Gannon." For the life of me, I could not figure out how to change it back and had to call him—yes, we had a telephone conversation about this. At that moment, we all were convinced that Gannon could read! Prior to this incident, the grandson we knew spoke very rarely, uttering just enough words to get his desires fulfilled. Now we saw that he had taught himself not only how to use the computer but also how to read.

And I was thrilled to have a computer guru in the family, as I am very inept when it comes to this technology. In fact, the next time I was at Gannon's house, I sat with him while he worked at his computer. I found it fascinating, but I guess I asked way too many questions, because he turned to me and very calmly said, "I really like you, but you're annoying me." Oops! I left the room.

Gannon continued to surprise us. One of the characteristics of PDD is that children on the spectrum drift into their own world and are unaware of those around them. Gannon's mom and dad were convinced he didn't even know he had a younger sister. But as a result of the many protocols he had been through, he began demonstrating significant progress. At the age of six, he "discovered" Ella. She is three years younger than Gannon, and she's a firecracker. She became a daily irritant in his young life, and he became one to her as well. Life became even more interesting.

One day after dropping Heidi off at a doctor's appointment, I took Gannon and Ella to lunch. Ella was acting up (nothing new), and even though she was only around three years old, she had quite a vocabulary. She was getting on Gannon's nerves and, quite honestly, on mine. Gannon asked her nicely to "SHUT UP!" I asked him not to use that word, and Ella, in a very authoritative voice, told him the same thing. They bantered back and forth until Gannon laid down the law by saying, "Don't talk back to me, young lady." (Wonder where he had heard that phrase?) Several days later, he asked Heidi if she was going to have another Ella. Heidi told him she didn't plan on having any more children, and he walked out of the room saying, "That's great!" Yep, he was well aware he had a little sister!

Gannon is also one of the bravest boys we know. He never complains, never says "no" to any of the protocols he is asked to do, the doctors he has to visit, the pills he has to take, his limited diet, or any of the other numerous requests made by his mom, dad, doctors, and teachers. He is a living embodiment of Ernest Hemingway's observation that courage is "grace under pressure."

And he continues to amaze us every day. He is winning his battle with autism. He is recovering! Heidi remains an outspoken advocate for autism awareness and, by example, so does Gannon. At the age of nine, he addressed a banquet room full of parents, educators, and physicians at an International Autism Conference to share his journey of hope. He received a standing ovation! And today, at the age of fourteen, he had one of the lead roles (the meerkat Timon) in his school's play *The Lion King, Jr.* His show-stopping performance of acting, singing, and doing comedy all while interacting with the other actors on the stage brought him his second standing ovation!

As his grandparents and staunch admirers, we also give Gannon a standing ovation for his courage, progress, achievements, superb attitude, and sense of humor. We wish him a future filled with many successes, which surely will come. For, after all, he is a child of God! We started this chapter with a scripture verse and would like to end with one as well:

"Do not be anxious about anything, but in every situation, by prayer and petition, with thanksgiving, present your requests to God." Philippians 4:6.

Patricia Swarthout
(Stepmother of Team TMR's Bling)

13

Moira

If I Knew Then . . .

WHEN I READ THE THINKING MOMS' REVOLUTION BOOK *EVOLUTION OF a Revolution: From Hope to Healing*, I was so moved that I cried through the first few chapters. I was amazed at the strength and determination of the mothers who fought so hard to figure out what had happened to their children. I finally understood what my daughter Meadow had been trying to tell me for years. (She wrote a chapter in the book.)

I was a teenager in the 1970s, when women's rights were huge and we were told we could do *anything* we wanted. My friends were going to college to obtain careers. I graduated with honors and also had the opportunity to go to college, but the summer after I graduated, I met my first real love and decided that what I really wanted was to be married and raise a family. So I was married at nineteen and had my first child, a beautiful little girl, a couple of months before my twenty-first birthday. I went on to have four more children during my fifteen-year marriage.

I had all of my children, two girls and three boys, by natural childbirth (no drugs), which was the preferred method back then. They all received their recommended vaccinations—yes, I was one of the sheep that didn't even question such things. The vaccine schedule in 1983 looked quite different from the schedule my grandchildren have today, however. According to the CDC website, the vaccination schedule for my children had been five doses of DTaP, five doses of the oral polio vaccine, as well as one dose of the MMR and Td vaccines. The vaccine schedule put out by the CDC for 2014 is six pages long, with many footnotes and variations. It lists ten additional types of vaccines; the current number of shots given before the age of eighteen is thirty-three (my kids received twelve).

My five children had the usual childhood illnesses, like ear infections and chicken pox, but nothing out of the ordinary. They all thrived and met their childhood milestones.

My oldest daughter, Meadow, is very bright and talented. She has always been mature for her age—we potty trained her at seventeen months. When Meadow was three years old, she and her sister attended ballet classes and preschool; they later also took piano lessons. Meadow excelled in school and was often chosen for singing solos in school concerts; she was also talented in art, winning competitions in grade school. In high school, she was a pompom girl and part of the show choir. She helped me take care of her younger sister and brothers and never caused any problems; she was an especially big help when I went through my divorce.

When Meadow was sixteen, she met the love of her life. She eloped at eighteen and moved to Texas, close to his family. I was devastated! I felt she had more to offer the world than just being a wife and mother. She made the same mistake that I had made: choosing to start a family at a young age instead of using her talents to have a successful career.

My first grandchild, a dear little boy named Tristen, was born when I was only thirty-nine. I remember Meadow telling me he was always sick with high fevers and ear infections. After they moved back to Wisconsin, I had a chance to observe him myself, and I remember that he only ate certain foods and loved lining up his trains. He had certain routines that had to be followed or he would get very upset. He was still getting sick all the time.

When Tristen was about fourteen months old, Meadow and I took him to Georgia to see his dad graduate from Basic Training. We stopped at gas stations and rest areas on the outskirts of towns so Tristen could get out of his car seat and run around. I remember that he was coping pretty well as long as we made those stops. On the way back to Wisconsin, however, I was feeling tired and just wanted to get home. So I stopped at a gas station in the middle of a busy town instead of looking for one on an off-ramp. Meadow got Tristen out of the car seat, turned to get her purse, and he was off! I came around the car just as another car was backing up over him! Meadow screamed and tried to push the car off of Tristen. I peeked under the car, my heart in my throat, and saw little Tristen's blue eyes blinking back at me. I told the driver to pull forward and we grabbed Tristen. He had a burn on his arm from the tailpipe, but otherwise he was unharmed. IT WAS A MIRACLE! I knew that God had blessed us and that Tristen was a special spirit meant to be in this world.

Through his first years, Meadow studied Tristen's habits and wrote a paper on his behaviors to show the doctor when she went to him with her concerns. The doctor was so impressed that he asked for a copy to show to other parents. At two years old, Tristen had no language, so he was given a hearing test, which he passed. He was then referred to Early Intervention Services.

Just after his brother Tanner was born in 2000, Tristen was diagnosed with PDD-NOS and a fever of unknown etiology. At four years old, he was diagnosed with a sleep disorder. At eight years old, he was diagnosed with autism and had tubes put in his ears.

Meadow researched autism tirelessly, started her own blog, and joined the Thinking Moms' Revolution community. She also became a paraprofessional for special needs children.

I remember reading one of my daughter's blog posts about how alone she felt and how everyone around her (she had moved to a new area) thought her ideas were crazy. The post made me cry, and I realized what a strong and special person she was to go with her instincts and beliefs on what was best for the health and healing of Tristen and her family no matter what other people thought. I am so grateful she found TMR and the support of other mothers going through the same challenges.

Meadow has tried many therapies, including yeast treatment, Lyme treatment, chelation, infrared sauna, HBOT, chiropractic therapy, and speech therapy. Whether she was in a nearby town or far away, she always called me to tell me of his progress. I remember how excited she was when he started sharing memories of when he was little, and the first Christmas he showed real joy and wonder as he opened his presents. I also remember the difference in Tristen when he switched to a gluten/dairy-free diet—he no longer lay on the floor and cried when things didn't go his way or got overwhelmed by the environment of family gatherings.

Meadow is the go-to person in our crazy, mixed-up family. She is always kind and caring, but firm in her beliefs and morals. I now realize she was not fated to be a famous artist or musician; she was meant to be exactly who she is and do exactly what she does. Her purpose in life has been to help her son be all that he can be, to help her whole family be healthier, and to make a difference in the world through sharing her beliefs and experiences. Meadow has never treated Tristen any differently than she would any other child, setting boundaries and rules for his behavior to help him adjust. The rest of our family also never treated him differently; we all love and accept him.

One day, Meadow hopes to open a home for special needs children and run it with the knowledge she has acquired through her experience and research. And I know she can do it! For now, she continues to push that two-ton weight off of Tristen and heal him, while also working to educate others.

All that my daughter has gone through with Tristen and shared about his healing led me to do my own research. I started wondering about my youngest son, who was much more difficult to raise than my other children had been.

When I was pregnant with him, I already knew my marriage was over. I was working full time, and I was under terrible stress from the problems in my marriage, but I knew I had to take care of this special baby growing inside me. When the doctor told me I had gestational diabetes, I changed my eating habits from junk-food snacks to carrot sticks, raisins, and sunflower seeds. I ate salads for lunch. I also decided to go with a nurse-midwife for the birth. My husband was always gone, so I did everything on my own, including caring for my other four children.

T was born a healthy baby boy. He gave me something positive to focus on and the strength to go through with my plans to file for divorce. The divorce process would become one of the worst experiences of my life. I cannot even explain the horrific stress my husband put me through. At one point, I got in my car and started driving towards Idaho, where my sisters lived. I was obviously out of my mind (now that I look back on it), but all I kept thinking at the time was that I had to get away. Realizing I couldn't leave my children behind, I turned around in Minnesota and came back. With my parents' help, I was able to move into my own place when T was one year old.

I cannot describe the peace I felt when I held my baby in my arms in the rocking chair in my new home. I had five children to care for while working full time, and I wasn't sure how we were going to buy food . . . but I was free! Thank goodness for Meadow, who was always there to be supportive and help with whatever I needed. She even made the move to a new town with me when she was sixteen, leaving her school, all her activities, her friends, and an offer from her dad to buy her a car if she moved in with him instead.

I never noticed any specific regression in T. He seemed to be a normal, happy, healthy toddler, though I did have a difficult time potty training him, which had been a breeze with all my other kids, and he continued to need Pull-Ups at night. I was concerned but thought he would outgrow it. Then, when he went to preschool, I started getting reports of bad behavior from T's teachers, who said that he wouldn't listen, participate, or cooperate.

At the time, I was working a second job on weekends and my other daughter, who was seventeen, watched him for me. I would come home from work to find he had spray painted the garage or brought stray kittens into the house. One time he had even set the carpet in my bedroom on fire. I quit my second job to spend more time with him and supervise his activities.

When T was in the first grade, he wasn't cooperating with the teachers or participating in activities, and he was getting more and more violent. I was constantly called to the school, as T was having fits, screaming, and throwing desks. He absolutely refused to do anything during his swimming class once he got in the water. This was a kid that loved going to the beach with us when he was a toddler . . . I couldn't understand it. During this time, T had a really good counselor who met with me and did his best to work with my son. Unfortunately, he wasn't very successful.

I was so upset. I just did not know what to do. I realized that life was difficult after my divorce and there was a lot of stress brought on by my ex-husband, but T had so much family around him that loved him. I begged him to tell me what was bothering him, but he just kept saying he didn't know.

Back at this time, the big diagnosis for kids with behavioral problems was ADHD. I heard about it and was so desperate to find something that would help him. I took him to his doctor, who diagnosed T with ADHD. He didn't do any tests or ask me to further monitor him; he just listened to my descriptions and prescribed Ritalin. I didn't even own a computer back then, so I just read the pamphlets the doctor gave me and trusted that he knew what he was talking about.

T hated the Ritalin; he said it made him feel sluggish and spacey. He also attended counseling and therapy, but all that he learned from these was how to stifle his anger. My ex-husband blamed me for T's behavior, saying I must have been drinking or taking drugs while I was pregnant. I never drank or used drugs during any of my pregnancies; I did not even smoke cigarettes, as many did back then. I was still consumed by guilt, however, because I was sure that the stress I was under during and after the divorce had somehow caused T's psychological damage.

As an adult, T still deals with anxiety and depression; he also continues to stifle his anger. He loves me, his dad, and his family, but he does not like people in general and prefers to be alone. He has a job and lives with a roommate but spends most of his time in his room by himself. He is very good-looking and has had several opportunities for relationships, but he doesn't have a girlfriend because he fears intimate relationships. He talks to me a lot and expresses his feelings and fears, and it breaks my heart that I cannot do more to help him.

How I wish I had had a support group like TMR when T was a child! Maybe something as simple as a change in diet would have helped him. With all I've learned from my daughter and *Evolution of a Revolution: From Hope to Healing*, I no longer believe T's problems are purely psychological. I believe that the stress during my pregnancy could have caused some damage, but I also believe that there are ways to help my son that do not involve prescribed medications. When did we become a nation where every behavior has a label (OCD, PTSD, MDD, Bipolar, etc.) and a medication to "cure" it?

My daughter recommended a natural supplement for T called 5-HTP, which helped with his depression, but I cannot get him to take it regularly, as he still hates pills. I am hoping that I can use my new knowledge to convince him to look into natural healing methods, but it is hard to make sure he follows through when he is an adult living on his own.

I firmly support my daughter's beliefs, and not just because I have seen the difference they have made in Tristen's life. I have also seen the benefits to her entire family. When I was a young mother, I also wanted to do the best I could for my children. I read Dr. Lendon Smith's *Feed Your Kids Right*. I tried a no-refined-sugar diet (I used fructose back then). I made homemade all-grain breads. I had a huge garden and grew and preserved my food. On the farm we raised a pig, Angus cows, and free-pecking chickens for our meat. As life got more complicated and stressful, I had to struggle just to survive, and I became overwhelmed and focused just on getting through each day. I wish things had been different, but I can do nothing but go forward from here.

I believe my daughter when she tells me she has discovered something new and continue to be amazed at her strength and fortitude. After reading the stories of the brave mothers of children with autism, I felt the need to warn some of the young girls at work about vaccination dangers. One of the girls looked at me and smiled. I said, "What, you have heard about this?" She said, "Yes, and I've heard it's not true." Okay, Meadow, I get what you are up against!

Surprisingly, my girlfriends my age are much more open-minded and actually listen to what I have to say. I was stunned to find out that one of my friends, who has a granddaughter with autism, said she saw a regression in her after her twelve-month vaccinations. She said she believed the vaccinations caused this regression, but she could never find any proof. Sadly, the granddaughter died when she wandered away, fell into a swimming pool, and drowned.

I continue to tell my co-workers my daughter's story, and if they think I am crazy, then so be it. I can't help but hope to help at least one person. Revolution can be a slow process, especially when you are dealing with a nation of sheep who blindly follow what they are told. It takes strength, courage, and commitment to fight against the status quo.

After reading *Evolution of a Revolution: From Hope to Healing*, I firmly believe in the testimony of the parents of children with autism. I

I hope people will continue to read the book and be enlightened. I hope it will instill in them the desire to become more educated on vaccine dangers and autism. I know it has inspired me, not only to share my own testimony of Tristen's journey to health, but also to look at how I myself can live healthier. Thank you, TMR, and thank you, Meadow, for bringing me into this fight. I hope that, as a "Thinking Grandmother," I too can help make a difference!

Jann Willard
(Mother of Team TMR's Green Bean Girl)

14

Rembrandt

What's on Your Resumé?

I PULL UP TO THE FRONT OF THE MIDDLE SCHOOL. HE GETS OUT OF the car, and as he walks to the front door with his aide, one free hand flies up to tap the bald spot at the back of his head. My heart sinks, and I wonder if I can get through the grocery store before I need to come back for him.

On June 3, 2002, Kiddo slid into the world faster than his doctor, midwife, mother, or I had expected. I reached out to stop him from falling off the bed and yelled for the nurse. In the scramble of "She has a while yet," "He's here!" and getting the medical staff to understand they needed to catch the doc before she left the building, we had been introduced to the way Kiddo's life would unfold. From that moment on, nothing was where it was expected to be, when it was expected to be, or especially how it was expected to be.

I'm a "baby boomer." Born in 1952, the eldest of seven, Scotch-Irish; both sides of the family included immigrants in the last two to three generations. Even though they had little formal education, they were smart, creative, and resourceful. Self-education and reading were a priority. They could make or fix anything and did their best to pass those skills on to kids and grandkids, pushing them to do well in school and aspire higher. We have family photos spanning five healthy generations. Though passing through Ellis Island involved undergoing physical and mental tests and getting doused with chemicals supposed to decontaminate and more, my people got through the ordeals with flying colors. They were part of the fabric from which America was built. They were part of the railroad, telephone, and manufacturing industries. They learned about finding a niche and going from having little to a solid middle-class life.

There were many changes that followed and brought Kiddo to where he is. Subtle changes, generations in the making. His great-great-great-grandfather grew food and was a greengrocer for the Great Atlantic & Pacific Tea Company for many years. He practiced organic farming on his oversized lot in Westfield, New Jersey. His wife cooked everything from scratch and taught three generations after her to do the same. My parents' generation didn't follow that practice—too many kids. Both of my parents ended up working one or more jobs, and the convenience foods crept in. When I was little, we were outside a lot to play, but being Scotch-Irish, we needed to be careful to avoid getting sunburned. Because of safety concerns, having working parents meant spending even less time outside. TV, while forbidden until the homework was done, was only too happy to fill the gap. Vitamin D wasn't even on the radar as a known cornerstone to long-term health. One A Day vitamins were supposedly all that we needed to be healthy.

Other things were changing too. The "Garden State" became a manufacturing center, filled with pollution and chemical dumping. Waterways became the vehicle for distributing poisons and toxins of all kinds. Farmlands began using chemicals, and the runoff added to the pollution problem. Wood, metal, and other natural materials gave way to plastics. Cotton, linen, and wool gave way to rayon, nylon, and polyester. Mosquitoes, no longer controlled by the decreasing amphibian population, were sprayed with great clouds of insecticides that wafted through neighborhoods where children played. Homes were insulated and heated with coal and oil that spilled black smoke into winter skies and fireplaces that spilled white smoke and ashes. Both of them added carbon dioxide into the tighter, less ventilated homes. Pretty much everyone had at least one car spewing lead into the environment. Over time, we saw the rise not only of clusters of unusual cancers, but also clusters of autism. When a child's cord blood is tested today, over 200 chemicals are found, which include trace chemicals that have not been used for decades. This means that these chemicals are stored in the body fat of generations of women and passed down to their offspring.

What else was changing? Social structures and expectations were evolving fast. Television. JFK was killed. Vietnam happened. Civil rights and women's rights surged into public consciousness. Baby boomers were caught in the middle of all the changes. In the dialogue of what women could and couldn't do, what people of all races could and couldn't do, we acquired only a superficial semblance of self-determination. Given that women are still often presented as ignorant, stupid, hysterical, or unable to make a rational, common-sense decision, we know that that dialogue has not moved one inch in almost fifty years.

Losing trust has been a long process. The myth of the way the world is supposed to work has given way to seeing how it really does. Assumptions about family structures (such as the male head of the household being the steadfast and loyal Prince Charming) have come crashing down. The notion that women have acquired true self-determination because of "women's lib" has come crashing down. Everything else that was built on that idea of a stable family with roles assigned and met has come crashing down. So here we are, looking around, seeing what we thought was truth dissolve into myth. No, not every man is raised to be the wage earner and family support. No, women were not and are not allowed to choose a free life path. No, not everything at the grocery store is meant to nourish you. No, killing little things *can* harm big things (including people). No, the ocean is not bottomless. No, having a formal education does not make you an expert. No, having a license does not make you competent. No, the idea that modernity always means progress is not correct. No, being a grandma doesn't mean I get to bake cookies for happy little kiddos who sleep over on school vacations and get spoiled on birthdays and Christmas. At least not yet.

Oh sure, they sleep over, but it isn't always happy. Sure, I bake cookies after sifting through thousands of recipes with alternative ingredients. Sure, they get spoiled on birthdays and Christmas, but everything feels disconnected. The intended age on the box doesn't match the age, behavior, or developmental stage of the child. Here is a child between two and six years of age who doesn't know what to do with toys except dump them on his head because he has no understanding of the life experiences that cars and trucks represent. Here is a ten-year-old who is still attached to Thomas the Tank Engine and who will become a twelve-year-old shopping on eBay for toys he saw advertised in 2004 (my best guess is that 2004 is where he lost connections that we are trying to find). He lives with a fourteen-year-old sibling who doesn't ask for anything because his younger brother will take it or break it because he lacks the understanding that it doesn't belong to him.

It would be *so* easy to say it was the vaccines. So there he was, sliding into the world in 2002, and of course he had the hep B vaccine at birth, even though it doesn't show up on his record. He had colic, soft stools, and he cried a lot. He had the DTaP/IPV and COMVAX (Hib + hep B) shots at two months. That's when the first of the ear infections came. Colic continued, and he still needed a lot of holding and rocking. He didn't babble. He didn't make eye contact. DTaP, IPV, COMVAX, and PCV7 were all given at four months. His mom struggled with breast feeding, so we tried soy formula supplements.

Many ear infections, many antibiotics, chronic diarrhea; he struggled to sleep and was miserable when awake. Doctors were useless. I was still involved in my art career and did not experience firsthand what my daughter and her sons were going through because she lived out of town and we were only visiting a couple of times a month at best.

December arrives, and with it DTaP and IPV. My grandson has no inkling of what to do with toys, makes no eye contact, doesn't babble, screams unless he is held, and needs to be rocked to sleep. His big interest on Christmas Day is a tag hanging from a stuffed toy. Auntie holds him high on her shoulder so that her shoulder presses into his tummy. Something is clearly wrong, but the doctors don't have any answers. We have allergies in the family, but removing the usual suspects from his diet doesn't seem to make a difference. The ear infections are still constant. Antibiotic after antibiotic is prescribed.

My daughter and her boys are now living in town and I'm seeing more of them. They move and come back. Kiddo is still not responding like he should. May rolls around, and with it another round of DTaP, IPV, and COMVAX vaccines. He doesn't play; he dumps his toys on his head. When we pick them up, he grabs the bins and does it again. He still doesn't sleep unless rocked, sometimes for hours. Diapers are full of pasty poo and black sandy specks; the doctors put tubes in his ears because ear infections never clear up and the antibiotics are useless.

August 2003. Kiddo is fourteen months old, and he is given the MMR and chickenpox vaccines—while having yet another fever. We didn't yet know that a child with a fever should not receive a vaccine until he is well again! He gets the MMR twice actually, on the day of the fever and again the next time he is brought in to check his ears, because no note had been made of the first one. It's all over at this point. He stands on his head all the time. He screams for hours on end. It isn't close enough to the injection to blame the MMR vaccine, but the non-stop screaming lands him in the ER. They keep him, dose him with Valium, look for brain tumors to explain the screaming that doesn't stop for thirty-six hours. No tumors are found, and the docs just shrug. He's sent home and his mother is given antibiotics, and Tylenol, and Valium to shove down his throat. She has to sit over him to do this, pinning him to the floor. We are all helpless, though no one is more helpless than he is.

We already know it's autism when we ask to have an evaluation. Kiddo is eighteen months old, and in addition to all the other things he isn't doing, he is also not growing. At twenty-four months, the state team confirms what we know.

Between that eighteen-month visit and the diagnosis, a little miracle happens. I open up a search page on the computer and find Defeat Autism Now! I call the number. The very first video recordings of a DAN! Conference have been released. I pay the $60 fee and download the videos. I'm speechless, with tears running down my face, as I hear Dr. Krigsman describe my grandson's stools. I am stunned as Dr. McCandless lists things parents can do to help make up for what the kids are missing. I listen three times to Dr. Pangborn explain what supplements will help. The local food co-op has some of what they suggest, and we get started.

I go to the pediatrician and insist my grandson be tested for food allergies. Again, there is another miracle. She did not subscribe to what was referred to as the "DAN! protocol" in those days, but a colleague of hers had spoken about DAN! being helpful, so she runs routine blood tests. The overall IgG is just a little high, so she agrees to sign off on an IgG test. The local allergist, who had tested him for IgE, says that there is no evidence of any allergies. She doesn't want to do the test. The pediatrician prevails, and the test is run. The results show moderate to high sensitivity to *twenty-six* foods. I don't think anyone would be surprised to hear these are the foods he commonly eats and that the mushy sandy stool is Exhibit A of a wrecked gut. We pull some foods out. We pull more foods out. We pull out foods that didn't test positive, because now there is a clear reaction to them. We get to the bottom of the food sensitivities, and he says his first intelligible word, "bubbles," during a therapy session. And for the first time in his life, his ears are clear.

As days run into nights, and nights run into days, and days run into weeks, and weeks run into months, Kiddo's father is suddenly out of the picture. His mother can only find low-wage jobs because she didn't finish school and no day care in town will take care of this child who screams, bangs his head, and can't talk. Even though we are making steady but miniscule improvements as we add in supplements and tweak Kiddo's diet, we have a long, long way to go.

When we first moved to town, I worked as the Adult Services Director for the local agency serving adults with developmental disabilities. I know where this child will end up if he doesn't start getting help now. It was part of my job back then to give parents the talk about not living forever. My daughter needed to finish school. I was working toward my life's dream. I had become a watercolor artist, joined a successful artists' co-op, and was working to help a historic downtown in a small town survive despite the presence of a Walmart. My husband and I had invested in a commercial building to house the artists' co-op with the intention for it to be the cushion for our retirement. Instead, the sale of that building financed our efforts to begin healing our grandson.

I started taking care of Kiddo so my daughter could work and go back to school. I also read, researched, and attended conferences. I watched conference videos over and over, learned what might work for him, and tried various approaches. Little by little, he showed improvements. When we first started, he had no reflexes; he couldn't pull his foot away from a thorn or feel a mosquito bite. Instead of rocking, his night-time routine became an Epsom salt bath followed by lights out and learning videos with low volume. I massaged him to sleep. Over time, the massage and supplements worked! First one leg reacted when I tapped his knee; three days later the other responded as well! We literally danced with excitement the first time he scratched an itch!

He learned to play by having toys that matched those he saw in his videos, and I was able to teach him to copy what he saw on the screen. And it wasn't a "stim"—he was matching scenes and dialogues trying to learn words! Somewhere between the *Signing Time* videos and *LeapFrog: Letter Factory*, we were able to verify that he was actually reading. He was also able to respond to notes if we gave him closed-ended questions to which he had to respond by circling or filling in the blank. Being able to use note cards to ask him things or give instructions and have him respond was game changing. Finding a way to communicate was an amazing breakthrough!

He is now learning to build storyboards and add captions on the computer at school. He can type, and he uses the computer extensively, but we are still not at the point where he can use it to type or select icons to spontaneously communicate thoughts and feelings. Today, he is following a normal growth pattern, and he speaks, though still not conversationally. He is still greatly frustrated by speech and not being able to retrieve the words he wants to say. His diet is still greatly restricted, but he loves wholesome foods that parents with kids eating the standard American diet have been brainwashed to believe their kids won't eat.

So why did I say it would be "easy to say it was the vaccines"? I am saying that vaccines are not the *only* cause. They are the trigger on the loaded gun, no question, but our guy also came into the world poisoned by mercury. His mother had dental work done while she was pregnant. She happened to be on Medicaid at the time. Like tens of thousands of other young women, the only option she had was mercury amalgam fillings. His birth was fast, even though her contractions were not progressive. She was given Pitocin to control the bleeding. I find it interesting that both my mother and I were also given Pitocin when we were giving birth to stimulate contractions. Pitocin is a synthetic form of oxytocin, and Kiddo is given supplemental oxytocin. In short, my grandson was affected by a lot of factors, from the accumulation of toxins from all sides of the family and the increasingly toxic environment to the decrease in crucial natural vitamin D and essential nutrient intake. All of these have become one huge web of entanglement.

Most recently, we have been sifting through the genetic puzzle. This child has African American heritage and Ashkenazy heritage, along with the Scotch-Irish genes. Poor Vitamin D production and utilization occur more frequently in populations in all three regions of his origin.

Poor methylation is more frequent in Irish populations. Food intolerances he has show up frequently in these groups as well. We are up against low production of many crucial cofactors and enzymes, and the problem is exacerbated by toxic overload and direct immune assault. In short, the proverbial "genetic predisposition" in reality isn't a predisposition to "autism." It is a predisposition to being unable to handle everything that the world throws at him. The vaccines are a part of the problem, a huge mega-slam assault, but they are not the only part. In my opinion, just avoiding the mega-slam is not enough. We have to clean up our act overall. No more "a little here" and "a little there." That approach has resulted in the proverbial snowball that grows bigger and bigger as it careens down the mountain.

We have done a number of lab tests. We have switched to a special diet that includes supplements. We have done HBOT and auditory processing therapy, and we still have more to investigate and more to try. Puberty has hit, and the changes that come with it have driven us back to random head bashing and repetitive speech. Seizures? PANDAS? We don't know yet. The only blessing at the moment is that, after a ten-year wait, we are finally processing the paperwork for his state Medicaid waiver. Ten years. How much of a difference might it have made if it were there sooner? His mom is almost finished with her education. That means she will be able to afford to give him a decent standard of living, with medical insurance that can interface with his funded services.

However, it also means that she MUST have someone to help her and give her the space to work. Someone needs to be there when the boy tapping that bald spot can't get it under control, when the frustration over not being able to retrieve a word overcomes him and that tap on the back of the head becomes the front of his head smashing a window. There has to be someone who can travel with him and help him get what he needs.

Your children NEED you. Your grandchildren NEED you. They need sleep when they are exhausted; they need someone to do the laundry. They need someone to do the dishes, cook, and pack the freezer. They need a weekend away here and there. They need a safe place to leave their children for few hours as often as you can manage—every week if possible. They need you to call and ask what they need from the store when you are out running errands to save them a trip. They need someone to help them read and remember the research, someone to partner with at conferences, someone to go with them to the doctor and lab appointments and pay attention to the information being given.

They need you to not be a wimp! Grandmas, they need you to make liars of the people who say older women are incapable or too old to be of use! Grandmas, if you can remember who is sleeping with whom on your favorite soap, then you can memorize the methylation cycle; just repeat the lessons enough times. Grandpas, if you can memorize sports stats, you can memorize supplement schedules and help prep what the kiddo needs.

That is the message I want to give to those of you who expect to be grandparents, as well as those who already are. There may still be family members out there who know how to cook from scratch. Have them teach you and do it. Learn to grow food or learn to choose products that are as whole, and unprocessed, and naturally cultivated as possible. Start detoxing your own bodies. Teach your children how to do it. Nothing you have worked for is more important. One in seventeen of us grandparents has an affected grandchild. WE DID THIS. We let the poisons and toxins creep in. We were complacent. We trusted in the benevolence of the system, and it let us down.

Examine your priorities and think for yourself. Help turn back the clock on what caused this to happen to this generation of kids.

Above all, remember that your son or daughter, or their spouses, are not to blame. It doesn't matter if you like them or not. It doesn't matter if they live the way you want them to or not. It doesn't matter if they are the "good" son or daughter. It doesn't matter if they look or act like your ex. It doesn't matter if their child, your grandchild, with autism doesn't hug, kiss, or even look at you, because it isn't about YOU. What they have going on inside takes precedence over everything else. If you waste time trying to guilt-trip your kid, blame your kid, or feel sorry for yourself, you are not just wasting your breath, you are wasting precious time and energy that could be spent creating love and healing for everyone. Who cares if you can't stand your daughter-in-law? She probably doesn't think you're a peach either, but you can ask her to show you what laundry supplies to use and spend a couple hours doing a chore to help her out. Being the Laundry Witch is better any day than just being a witch, and you don't even have to talk to each other.

Grandpa, you are also not off the hook. It doesn't matter if that guy she married doesn't deserve your little princess. You aren't being any knight in shining armor for your little girl when you sneer and belittle the guy who is as up to his knees in this disaster as she is. While he or your son are busting butt in a job they hate for the insurance your grandchild needs, you can be the taxi driver, the errand runner, the handyman. You can be the one to take the car to the shop or drive the other kids to soccer practice or dance lessons. It doesn't matter if your new wife doesn't want to help; you need to. Scheduling time to help when your ex isn't there is doable, so do it. If you and your spouse are still together, then double-team the support. If you see something that needs doing, DO IT. Don't wait for someone else.

We are no one. What we did for a living doesn't matter anymore. The stuff we owned doesn't matter anymore. It is no longer about us.

If you allow a kid to suffer because you are complacent, or lazy, or just plain selfish, that will speak greater volumes about you when you are gone than how many gold watches you got from Acme Sales Co.

If you favor the family not affected by autism and exclude your affected family members, you are lying to the ones you favor. You are giving your favored ones a sense that they are immune to having children who could be affected by autism and spectrum disorders, when in reality they and their children are in the same line of fire. Insist that family BE family. Stick together and support each other. Accept nothing less from your other children.

When we started our journey, there were no websites, Facebook, or blogs. There were a few books and conferences. Today there is TMR, TACA, Generation Rescue, National Autism Association, and more. There are more doctors and practitioners being trained every year. There are webinars and conference videos. Many people our age have a grandchild on the autism spectrum. That means that many of your peers are just as stunned and unsure of themselves as you are (or were). Be an example for them too. Help them become educated and inform their kids. Help them help their grandkids.

One more thing. There are grandparents out there who, because of tragedy or circumstance, are raising kids on the spectrum on their own. They may not have a network either. Or they may have a network and offer to invite you in and help show you the ropes. Reach out if they are alone. Accept if they reach out to you.

These kids can improve. These kids can recover. We can stop more from being affected. Let's get this network going. The world we leave behind depends on it. There's work to be done and your resumé fits the job!

Victoria J. West
(Friend of Team TMR)

15

Shotgun
Riding Shotgun

IN THE SUMMER OF 2011, MY DAUGHTER COLETTE WENT INTO LABOR with her first child. Issues occurred just minutes after she received her epidural. We were informed by a super-freaked-out nurse that my daughter needed an emergency C-section because of low fetal heart tones.

Luckily, the procedure went well. Within the hour, my sweet baby Gunner was here. He was beautiful and perfect. We were all so excited to have a new baby to cuddle. I had other grandchildren, but they were already teenagers, so it was nice to have a round two. Gunner weighed nine pounds, and he was so cute. He hardly looked brand new; he looked more like he was a few weeks old.

Things were good, and we were all so excited to gather around Gunner and love him to pieces. Since we come from such a big family, he had no shortage of visitors. Family and friends alike came to see the baby, wish Mommy and Daddy well, and share parenting tips. I was happy to see them beaming with pride holding their sweet baby and excited for them to get home and settle into life. I felt like they were going to have this great life with their kid—you know, all suburban and picket fence-y.

Within hours of being released from the hospital, Colette started to have some abnormal swelling and then a migraine. She was unable to sleep that first night after returning home. She was unable to lie flat without coughing. Her older sister talked her into returning to the hospital to get checked out. They learned pretty quickly that things were more serious than they had expected. Every test under the sun was performed, and a lot of fancy pants suit types came in to assure them about the level of care she would receive. They said things like "We will get you through this." At that time, we were still not told what it was they were going to be "getting her through."

She was admitted into the hospital and put on oxygen, with no explanation of what was causing the swelling, migraine, and need for oxygen. The details are kind of hazy now with all that has happened over the last few years, but I believe we found out what we were dealing with the next morning. Cardiomyopathy (weakening of the heart muscle) and congestive heart failure was her diagnosis.

How did this happen? Earlier this week we were welcoming a baby into this world, and then boom! Our whole world turned upside down. We were informed that because of the severity of her heart condition, she would probably never regain normal function. She had a couple of procedures during that first year, and she was monitored more closely than she wanted to be by both her doctors and our family. It's hard, as a parent, to watch your child's health decline in what seems like an instant, to wonder what happened, what made your child sick. How will this pan out in the long haul? My daughter was twenty-five years old, with a new baby and a heart condition. I'm sure anyone reading this book can relate to the shock.

Gunner, meanwhile, hit all of his milestones on time; he went in for a well baby check when he was around sixteen months old. After this visit, things changed forever. He stopped responding to his name, and we were all convinced he was deaf. His parents took him back to the pediatrician within the week. It was decided that because of his frequent ear infections, it would be best if he went to an ENT. The ENT thought that tubes were needed to help him out and that Gunner should start responding and talking again. That didn't happen. As I mentioned earlier, Gunner was my daughter's first child, and he was the BABY of the family. We didn't want to see anything wrong, and, to be honest, we knew nothing about autism. NOTHING.

Colette could not shake the feeling that something was going on with Gunner, however, so she dove into Google and started researching his behaviors. She later approached all of us for support, looking for our opinions and input. I'm embarrassed to say that she didn't receive any support. No one else was ready to face Gunner's developmental delay. We all told her that she was being nuts and should get off Google and start getting out of the house a little more often. The pediatrician ended up agreeing with Colette, however, and referred Gunner to a developmental pediatrician. The wait time for an appointment is usually four months. In the meantime, Colette researched the gluten-free/casein-free/soy-free diet and decided to start Gunner on it. She also called Missouri First Steps and started him in Early Intervention Services.

I was also doing a lot of my research myself, though on the wrong websites. They suggested you accept your child's condition but offered no plan or hope of recovery. Why did I waste my time reading things that were not offering solutions and answers? I have no idea, but I'm glad that's behind me.

Dealing with the stress that autism brings into your life can be so hard. It affects every aspect of life. It changes you in a way you can't explain. Even before you get the official diagnosis, things are different. I was terrified and devastated for my grandson, for my daughter, and for us, his grandparents. We realized that our lives would never be the same. NOTHING would EVER be the same.

In June of 2013, when he was twenty-two months old, Gunner was diagnosed with moderate to severe autism. A few months later, he also received the diagnoses of hyperkinesis, encephalopathy, and, this year, epilepsy. It was hard on everyone, and I grieved for all of us. When he received his autism diagnosis, he had been receiving Early Intervention Services for around three months already. His therapies included special instruction, speech therapy, occupational therapy, applied behavior analysis, and hippotherapy. He was also in a research study with KU Medical, focusing on eye contact, social cues, and joint attention. He remained nonverbal. It was so difficult to look at this baby who had once been SO happy and SO healthy and not feel totally devastated that this was now his life.

I was angry that my daughter's family was suffering another blow and that once again the life I thought they would have was disappearing. I felt so hopeless. And to be honest, I was a negative part of Gunner's first year after he received his diagnoses. I didn't want my daughter to get her hopes up. I didn't want the family to be taken advantage of, because I knew they would do anything and spend every dollar they had and more to try to recover him. I could see the stress my daughter was putting on herself with all of Gunner's therapies, and I was anxious about how it was going to affect her health. I was afraid she would not see the results she so desperately wanted to see.

I am a mother; I always have my children's best interest at heart, even when it doesn't look that way to them. When my daughter immediately started Gunner on the GF/CF/SF diet—and when I say immediately, I mean the day she realized he had autism, before any doctor's appointments—she and I had a problem, because I didn't believe in the diet. I'm embarrassed to admit that I made things way harder on my daughter by questioning her and giving her the "tone." I was clueless. Looking back, I cannot believe that I was being so difficult because Colette had decided to put Gunner on an organic diet, free of gluten and casein. Really? I think I was just afraid it wasn't going to "work." I didn't want my daughter spending the extra money and stressing herself for nothing. I realize now that the diet did and continues to help him, and he just cannot have certain foods.

Gunner started feeling better, and the fog he had been living in lifted away. He could now look at us again. The eye contact was brief, but it was still progress. Before starting the diet, he also had a lot of stims and OCD behaviors. These behaviors decreased significantly within weeks of the diet changes, which took place before Gunner began any therapy.

Colette used the guide from the website of TACA (Talk About Curing Autism, a national organization dedicated to providing information, resources, and support) to get it all figured out. I became interested because I could see the improvements in his behavior—he seemed happier and more engaged. I did my own research and read what my daughter already knew. Certain foods are not processed by kiddos on the spectrum correctly, so they have the same effect as an opiate pill would.

I had a hard time adjusting to the new arrangements because the rules for my relationship with Gunner were different than the rules for all of the other children in my life. My daughter and I had it out a time or two over consistency. As a Nana, I wanted to spoil my baby Gunner. I felt that it was my God-given right as his Nana. This caused problems and stress for his parents. They were working so hard day in and day out with his therapists to help him, and we, the grandparents, were undoing hours of therapy work. We meant well, but it was hard for us to make Gunner use his words, so we would anticipate his needs and make sure everything went his way. If he wanted to stim, OK, let him stim on.

It took me a long time to acknowledge that I knew a lot about being a mother/grandmother to a typically developing child, but nothing about how to help raise a child with autism. Gunner's parents had to prove me wrong time and time again. I had to step back and realize that the three of them were literally fighting for their lives, and I had to trust that they knew best. Does fighting for their lives sound dramatic? Well maybe to some, but it really isn't an exaggeration. They were working hard every day in therapy, in their home program, with doctors, and with supplement regimens to help heal Gunner. That's the goal of this family, and it's our job as part of the family to help in whatever way we can. We have to believe that recovery is possible for all of them, but especially for Gunner. He deserves to live a life free of pain, to be able to share a belly laugh with a friend, to drive a car, to get married and have a family of his own. He deserves the life we all envisioned for him before autism came into the picture.

My advice to grandparents would be to trust your children. I learned this from experience. Colette and Travis are smart, and they are great parents. They both love Gunner to the moon and back. I know they do their research, and I know they won't try a new treatment unless they feel confident that it will help my Gunny bunny. It is no longer my job to guide my daughter on parenting because, really, I have no idea how to raise a child with autism. It's my job to support their decisions. It's my job to love Gunner and to love my daughter, not to question her judgment.

I have seen the results of her judgment firsthand. The progress Gunner has made in a little over a year is incredible. I no longer see a sad, tired, frustrated baby. He's a happy little boy, and he is becoming quite the chatterbox. He is doing so many things that mainstream doctors said would not be in the cards for him, even with intensive therapy interventions. I believe that all of these things are happening because of persistence. Gunner's parents never accepted that limited life for him, and I know they never will. They will continue to fight for him. Recovery happens every day, not because some people get lucky, but because they treat every aspect of the autism. AUTISM IS MEDICAL. It is not a brain disorder; it is a whole body disorder, and you have to treat all of the underlying conditions as well.

I'm so thankful that Gunner's parents stuck with the diet and added in the biomedical treatments. I am always leery when they start something new, but each new treatment brings more gains. Gunner started the Speak supplement in May, and within days he was singing songs! They started probiotics and a yeast treatment a few months ago, and we saw more big gains. He has always had a big sensory diet, and they even built him a sensory room in their home. Does it come cheap? No! Is it easy? No! Is it extremely stressful on them all the time? Yes. But it's worth it. He is worth it.

When Gunner was first diagnosed, I didn't see the life we have now. I saw sadness. I saw a sick little toddler in his own world, unable to connect with those who loved him dearly. I saw him crying and lashing out because he could not communicate. I'm so happy to let other families know there is hope, real hope. I see it every day in Gunner, as he is overcoming all of his obstacles.

When he was first evaluated for Early Intervention, he could not point, he could not look you in the eye, he had no speech, and he no longer played with any toys appropriately. To put it simply, Gunner had lost all of his skills. His regression took everything. The only things that remained were autism behaviors and stims. Fast forward to today, and Gunner is excelling in pre-K skills. He is no longer considered nonverbal, he can communicate his needs and wants, and he even gives us a sweet "I love you." A few weeks ago at school, a classmate was upset and crying, and Gunner reached out and rubbed the boy's back, saying, "It's okay." A child that not long ago couldn't care less if someone else were in the room was now trying to comfort a friend.

Recovery doesn't happen overnight. It's not a single transformation. It's a million little things happening as symptoms slowly disappear. As I sit here and write, it's hard to pinpoint specific examples because there are so many, and they all seem so small individually. But when put together, the changes are powerful. It is comforting because Gunner's quality of life is so much better. I don't want to jinx him, but I feel that he's well on his way to recovery and that one day he will lose that diagnosis.

We often say there are some things about Gunner that we hope never go away, like the belly laughs he lets out while playing fetch with the dogs, how excited he is to help me go to the chicken coop and collect the eggs, or how much he loves watching a helium balloon bounce off the ceiling. I love the ornery grin he gets on his face when he decides to do something he isn't supposed to do.

I would never ever in a million years say I am thankful for autism, because I am not! I hate autism, I hate the stress it has put on my daughter, and I hate that my grandson was and is sick! I hate that it has snatched time from us. I hate that Gunner is only three and has already had to endure so much, and that he has to work so hard in therapies. But I'm thankful that we have found other parents who have recovered their children, and that they are sharing their stories and helping guide younger children like Gunner onto that path to recovery.

I feel in my heart of hearts that Gunner will make it out to the other side. Recovery is possible; we will all keep working and keep fighting every day until he gets there. I feel much better now that I have found my role. I'm riding shotgun on this ride. I am not the driver. I can still make suggestions, but no one likes a backseat driver. I feel that for our family, things work better if I allow his parents to have the wheel. They know what needs to be done, they are living it, and planning out the next move, as well as the backup plans for the backup plan at 4:00 a.m.

To question your child's well-researched plan of action is hurtful. Even though you aren't saying they don't have their children's best interest at heart, and even though you aren't saying, "Don't try that, you are being nutty," that's how it will feel to them. Just realize that they have to think about the big picture, and that what may seem to you like innocent Nana spoiling may actually be confusing your grandchild if they have trouble generalizing. The mixed messages could cause a meltdown later or make them act inappropriately in another social situation.

When my daughter was in high school, around graduation age, I loved the song "I Hope You Dance" by Lee Ann Womack. I remember giving my daughter the CD. I heard it the other day, and I realized that the song still applies. I think maybe she took some of it to heart. The second verse especially.

I can't say enough how proud I am of her or how much I love my Gunny Bunny. Colette, thank you for teaching me to become a more patient and understanding mother and grandmother. When others saw mountains, you saw recovery. Most importantly, thank you for helping Gunner to dance.

Penny Canchola
(Friend of Team TMR)

16

Za Za

My Journey with Carmine

AUTISM. SEVEN YEARS AGO, IT WAS A WORD THAT I BARELY UNDER-stood. I had heard of autism, but I knew nothing about it. Well, I know much more now, and I am learning more every day. It has completely changed my life. As I write this, our grandson will soon turn seven. He is the most beautiful boy, with his bright blue eyes and his constant smile! Thank you, Lord!

Our grandson's name is Carmine. Our daughter, Tara, was on her own with Carmine by the time he was two months old. She moved six hours away from us so that she could find work. I would go to their home to visit or they would come to our place. Sometimes he would stay with us for a week at a time.

During the times that he stayed with us, I would say words to him so that he could try to repeat them, just like I did with my own kids when they were young. But it seemed he could not repeat sounds or small words in a way that we could recognize. For instance, the word "boo" would come out sounding like "baa." At first, I thought his hearing was impaired, but his hearing test came back perfect. I think that, for me, this was the first indication that something was very wrong. My grandson was nonverbal, even though I could tell he understood everything we said to him.

He also didn't seem to care whether he ate or not. This really stressed me out. How could a child have no appetite at all? How was he going to grow and be healthy? I had never experienced anything like this with my kids and knew nothing about it. I finally looked on the Internet and found out that there were many children with feeding issues. Of course, this was before he was diagnosed, so I did not know much about what eating and sensory issues were. The actual term is "feeding disorders." In Carmine's case, he was not interested in eating and seemed to be unable to chew food. So his food had to be soft so that he could just swallow it without chewing. He was hand-fed like an infant, and he would try to refuse the food. There was a constant battle to make sure he would get enough to eat every day.

As time went on, we saw that other skills were not coming along as they should have been. When it came time to try walking, he would not try the typical way. Most children will pull themselves up on the furniture and hold on as they walk along. He did not do this. He would not let us help him by holding his hands and balancing him on his feet. Then one day he just got up and started walking!

He was also not talking. He did not even try to copy words or sounds that he heard us say. He did not try to hold a crayon or focus on the paper so that he could try to draw or color.

Tara kept researching. She took Carmine to every doctor she could find. Then the seizures started. Small ones at first, but scary enough for someone watching their child go through them. Then Carmine had more serious seizures that nobody could explain. The doctors had called his small seizures "febrile seizures," even though he never had a fever with them. These new seizures were completely different. They started after he received his Hib vaccine, hepatitis A vaccine, and flu shot all at the same time.

Of course, Tara was alone with Carmine at the time it first happened. It was nighttime, and she had gone in to check on him before she went to bed. He looked catatonic, and his breathing was shallow. She called 911. The EMTs arrived, stabilized him, and took him to the hospital. By the time they arrived at the emergency room, Carmine was awake and seemed to be okay; he just wanted to sleep. Nobody could figure it out. The same thing happened again, with the same outcome. Nobody could even tell Tara what kind of seizure it was, or whether it even was a seizure, though the EEG testing showed that there was seizure activity. The neurologist wanted to put Carmine on medication, but that was too risky because it could have caused more seizures.

By the age of three, Carmine was walking but not talking. He was still only eating soft food that was hand-fed to him. He also did not use his fine motor skills for picking anything up. He scooped the object up instead. Tara was starting to suspect autism because she had been doing so much research, so she had him evaluated, and Carmine was diagnosed with autism. Tara found therapy for him, but nothing was really working. She felt that the mainstream medical profession was not giving her any answers. She felt they were letting her down and just leaving her to get through this alone. So she reached out to someone who told her about a naturopath that specialized in children with autism. She made an appointment. She soaked up all the information like a sponge, changing Carmine's diet and adding supplements. Financially, this really took a toll, but what a difference it made. He started being a little more verbal and focused, and he has not had a seizure in three years!

During all of this, Tara was trying to work and take Carmine to a daycare that was willing to feed a toddler by hand and change him as needed, as he was not potty trained. It was like taking care of an infant. Then she would pick him up and take him to preschool and doctor's appointments. It was too much. I was so afraid she would either have a complete breakdown or get very ill from the stress—she was getting sick every time our grandson came home with a runny nose. After four years, the time had finally come. Tara and I talked about making a drastic change. She made the decision to quit her job, and they moved in with us so that we could help.

We had moved to a new town due to changing jobs, so we rented a big house that would accommodate all of us. She took a year off work. It was a risk. She was adamant about being independent, so leaving a well-paying job was very scary. After they moved, Carmine was put into applied behavior analysis (ABA) therapy. He also needed intense feeding therapy.

Thank God for the university here! They have a wonderful special education program. After Tara got in touch with the professor in charge of the special education department, she helped us teach Carmine to at least not refuse the food when we tried to feed him. That was huge for us. It always used to be such a battle to get him to accept food, and Tara had tried so hard to avoid using a feeding tube. So far, she has succeeded, but at a huge cost. There is a lot of work that goes into preparing food for breakfast, lunch, dinner, and two snacks. Carmine still does not chew, so the food has to have the right consistency so that he can just swallow it.

We have been fortunate to receive other kinds of help from the special education department as well. We now have a wonderful group of students that are choosing special education as their major. They help with watching Carmine after school or babysitting when needed. I am so thankful for the network of people we have found here.

But the challenges continue too. We wanted to get Carmine potty trained and eating on his own before Tara went back to work. Well, that did not happen. They were living with us for two years, and he still is being fed by hand; we are also still working on the potty training. He understands how to do it but is very opposed to actually doing what is requested of him. So that is also a challenge.

Tara and Carmine have their own place now. I go over every morning to feed him breakfast, make his snack and lunch for school, and get him on the bus. The afternoons are usually covered by someone else, but I fill in when they are sick or cannot make it.

What I have learned about autism is this: it is a whole different world and people that are not in the midst of it have a difficult time understanding the frustration, the pain, the fatigue, the sadness. It takes a whole network of people to help, especially for a single parent. I watch our beautiful daughter immerse herself in getting her son well so that he can have a good life. I watch her never give up, even through all the stress of being a single parent and providing for both of them. I know how exhausting it is. I watched her stay at home every night for years, never giving a thought to her own life, and I worried because she was still so young and missing so much. That is probably the most difficult part for me as a parent. We all want the best for our children. We also want the best for our grandchildren.

In the end, though, Carmine has brought a whole new dimension to our lives, and a whole new set of people that we probably never would have known had it not been for him. We have learned so much about health and how certain things in our environment affect us. We will learn more.

I also learn from other parents and families going through similar situations. It helps to know that we are not alone. It gives me hope and inspiration when I read their stories and know that others are feeling the same as I do, and that some children have recovered. Autism seems to touch so many lives. There is an epidemic, and I want to scream because I feel sometimes that no one is listening. In light of the news from the CDC whistleblower, Dr. William Thompson, I feel very angry. He released a statement admitting that he and his colleagues at the CDC omitted information from a 2004 pediatric study which showed that African American boys were much more likely to be diagnosed with autism if they received the MMR vaccine before thirty-six months of age. The current vaccine schedule calls for children to get their MMR vaccine by the age of twelve months. That is when Carmine received his MMR vaccine.

What if all this could have been avoided? I think of our grandson and I think of all the thousands of children, parents, grandparents, aunts, uncles, and cousins out there experiencing the same things we do every day. It saddens me and angers me at the same time. I feel that the only people listening are the ones going through this. Finding the cause needs to be our priority. Why isn't it our government's priority?

I do know we will never give up helping him and trying whatever it takes to make him well. So much more needs to be done. More people need to hear these stories. Until Carmine and Tara came to live with us, I really did not understand the full extent of what goes on in a household with an autistic child: the everyday routines, the stimming, the repetitions, the meltdowns, all the food preparation, the expenses. The caregiver feels they could go crazy with it all. The ups and the downs. What an emotional rollercoaster! You want to give up on the recovery process and know you just cannot do that. Keep going. Keep hoping. Keep learning more and more. Keep trying.

To help me get some perspective on all that I was learning, I tried to find ways to understand and relate to what Carmine was going through. I remembered how I felt when my mother passed away. I was only eight years old. I remembered feeling so alone. I withdrew from people and became a very introverted child. I was also diagnosed with rheumatic fever after my mother passed away, so I could not go to school and had to be tutored at home. It was very lonely for an eight-year-old. Comparing our experiences, I started thinking that Carmine must feel very alone because he did not have words to let us know how he felt or what he needed.

I remember that being around animals helped me so much. We had horses, and it was wonderful therapy for a lonely child. Carmine also loves animals, so I felt we had something in common. Tara found a wonderful organization here that provides therapy using horseback riding. I have been lucky to take him to his weekly rides and watch him smile from ear to ear when he gets on that horse.

Carmine is so fortunate in that he has a loving and dedicated mother. He also has a wonderful grandpa (Papa), and a grandma, and an uncle who love him very much. Oh yes, and a Hurley dog (his uncle's) that he adores! He has a wonderful network of people around him, including other family members who have always been there for him and always keep him in their prayers. This is the hardest work I have ever done or seen done. But we will all keep on working and pushing on for his sake.

It helps that we are in the same town. We can lend a hand and be there when needed. Plus, it is great to watch our grandson grow and make progress. This progress is slow, but at least we are seeing it!

When Carmine was very little, he mostly babbled, but we noticed that he kept saying, "Za Za." It didn't sound like a word, so we could not figure out what it meant. Then finally one day Tara said, "I think he is calling you Za Za." Sure enough, every time he saw me, that was what he said. So it became part of our vocabulary. Now he can say Grandma, and that is so wonderful to me. He can even say, "I love you Grandma." I love, love, love it! But I feel I will always be Za Za, because it is so special that he found a way to give me a name when he had no other words. Sometimes I say "Za Za" to him and he looks at me and smiles!

Thank you so much, TMR, for this opportunity to be able to tell my story. It gives all of us a voice! It has definitely been quite a journey so far, and it continues on. God Bless you!

Jeannine Severns
(Friend of Team TMR)

17

Tiger Lily
Song of Sweetwater

Grandchildren

My munchkins, my puppies,
my television addicts,
helpless inside your videos
like butterflies under glass.
Your mother has left you
by a blue field of red rabbits.
She is too busy
with that beehive of an Internet
sucking out her own fable
of love and loss.
The screen buzzes and crackles
in its cage, my little pretties,
but don't be afraid.
Someday I will come

on my winged bicycle
and carry you off—
two Totos in a basket.

It's a hot August day, the weekend before my grandson Joshua's seventeenth birthday. He's a handsome young man, five feet five inches tall, with light brown hair and mesmerizing green eyes. Josh, as he prefers to be called, is at his computer, when he calls out to me from his room, "Grandma, come and see what's on my computer." The call is followed by raucous laughter. He shows me a video of SpongeBob removing his friend Patrick's head so he can't speak anymore. This scene is as familiar to me as my own face. Every day is like the movie *Groundhog Day*, a constant replay of the same scene. It's a symptom of his autism (which includes OCD and PANDAS) and one of the most obvious signs of his disability, though he also has cognitive issues and a social behavioral disorder.

When my daughter, Josh's mother, was five, she told me that someday she'd buy a house next to mine so I could be her babysitter. A prophetic remark, because I would later morph into her child's mother and father. Grandparents are supposed to visit grandchildren once a week to spoil them and flood them with gifts, aren't they? Josh moved in with me when he was eight.

I think back to the day Josh was born. Our family's joy was palpable. He was our first grandchild. He was healthy, the essence of perfection in our eyes. However, the euphoria was short-lived.

Like a brand new boat that sinks for unknown reasons, Josh's health deteriorated in the following weeks, and we had no answers. He suffered from reflux, persistent diarrhea, and lack of sleep; he cried all the time. He also had to fight pneumonia, RSV, ear infections, and asthma. My dream of taking an African safari quickly dissolved as I was sitting in a faux leopard-skin chair outside a hospital room. Josh was put on antibiotics for 151 days of his first year. He never missed any mandated vaccinations.

My love for him was boundless, but I was unable to stop the litany of ailments. He was clearly in pain. I rocked him, walked him, and drove him up and down the freeway at night so he could sleep. From that time forward, I became as indispensable as morning coffee, and my lifestyle changed as quickly as mercurial stars. I was no longer able to paint on canvas or socialize with friends. Instead I babysat Josh and researched autism.

When I needed a release from my own mental anguish due to my inability to resolve his disorder, I went home and wrote poetry, never realizing that it would be so difficult to write about illness because it generates too much emotion.

Slow Season

It's the slow season for words
each a frozen, veiny leaf
each a drop of blood on paper
cold as marble
She should have held the words
from the last winter's thaw
like an infant
when something seemed important

Despite his health problems, Josh was growing. He walked at nine months and used several words at a year. Newly divorced and temporarily unemployed, I devoted many hours to his care. So many, in fact, that I often felt overworked and underappreciated, though I never lost my sense of humor:

Daughter and Son-in-Law

They expect you to drop your life
as you would a stack of shirts

at the cleaners, then press you
to provide a two-hour service
unspotting their steamed up lives.
They spin their rack of power
like a roulette dealer.
Lady, they've got your number.
The baby's low on diapers,
a crisis of the derriere
You, fuming from all the crap
answer their call like a 911.
Your life, condensed into
an airtight bag, theirs
a storehouse of open containers.

Josh was diagnosed with autism before his third birthday, but there were signs of trouble by age two. His once agreeable temperament plummeted as fast as a downhill skier. His behavior became rigid and repetitive. He was hyperactive. Nothing seemed to please him. I combed the Internet for information and read a dozen books on autism.

Joshua

We applaud your birth,
a repetition of firsts,
child, grandchild,
cribbed in your gene pool
like a lobster in a fish tank.
Twenty digits intact,
perfectly shaped head,
your mouth round as a cheerio.

The next years turn over
like a capsized trawler.

Sickness snares
your ears, lungs, gut
with merciless frequency.
Vaccines boost insult.

Please stop screaming.
Tell us where it hurts.

We probe your lips for words.
All hesitation. Some days
phrases crawl out
in waves of duplication,
go adrift the next.
Where are you going?
Where are you going?
Your right eye's a glassy eel
swimming in that icy sea of autism.

Weeks after Josh's diagnosis, I flew to Washington, DC, where I attended my first conference, run by the National Vaccine Information Center. For two days, I felt submerged in my own tears. I saw videos of young children before and after they had been vaccinated. They had once been normal and healthy and then regressed into autism within weeks or months of the injections. Tots turned into sickly shells of their former selves. My grandchildren were never vaccinated again. Like so many others before me who drove along the same freeway, I now knew the exit that could alter the outcome.

Vaccine Injured

It was a calendar
of seasons realized

that left us
without illusions.
Joshua wouldn't be fine.
We backspaced
through time
to piece together
the ragged photos
of his primal years
inexplicable to those
who haven't
traveled here.

At three, his speech
simply echoes of echoes.
Words dangled
like dust in the air
of no meaning.
So he went inward
like a tortoise,
nobody could reach him.
But anger stalked
abruptly as whiplash.

He whacked toys, windows,
head banged into walls.
This side of autism
rooted in repetition
like the cookie moon,
he ate the same food,
watched the same video,
drew the same circle.
No one escaped.

Weeks turned into months. Josh's parents divorced and his mother returned to college. When his parents were unavailable, I became his primary caregiver. I took him to a Defeat Autism Now! (DAN!) doctor for medical help. In addition, he received applied behavior analysis therapy, a learning intervention to improve social and cognitive behaviors, speech therapy to increase his vocabulary, and occupational therapy to improve his fine motor skills. The schedule was rigorous; the gains were slow, but visible. Then, like an unexpected birthday gift, hope came dressed in autism ribbons. I joined the coterie of advocates who, like me, participated in fundraisers and political activism to place increased focus on autism and end our children's suffering.

Song of Sweetwater

"So what," you may say when I tell you
that while I'm on my way to pick up
my grandchild for speech therapy
two tires hiss like dissonant felines,
lower my car to the pitched pavement.
Only one spare and I can't change it.

My guess is you believe I'm lucky
to stall near the Sweetwater Church,
its spire rising like a coloratura's scales.
Neither tear nor prayer can summon a savior.
I'm the solo in the chorus of life
Thursday afternoon at a house of worship.

I think about my five-year-old grandson,
his voice stuck in that void of autism,
who recently held one note of
"You Are My Sunshine"
long enough to call it a song.

The autism community became the leading ensemble in my discordant world. I joined organizations to fight alongside others seeking answers to questions about autism's causes and cures. I frequented rallies, fundraisers, and conferences, often taking Josh, sucking up new information like a baby with a pacifier.

It's been an odyssey of highs and lows. There is no wizardry involved in autism. All of Josh's therapies have been helpful, but his biomedical treatments have contributed the most to his improvements. I found a new doctor, a functional medicine specialist, whom we still retain to this day. Together we work to enhance Josh's health and behavior by altering the gut microbiome, which directly affects what his brain can process. He has made tremendous progress over the years. He reads well, writes, has many friends, and is becoming more independent. He takes a truckload of supplements to boost his immune system, as well as prescription medicines when needed. Because his body is as porous as pumice stone, he is always susceptible to new bacteria, viruses, and parasites, which must be treated.

Josh is now in a tenth-grade special education class. He loves swimming, baseball, bowling, his laptop, and GF/CF chicken nuggets.

My days are now focused on Josh and the autism movement in general. However, I've also learned that, as a grandmother raising a young person, I need to be mindful of my own health, both mental and physical. I exercise by walking every day, seek out social activities, and maintain a nutritious diet. It's difficult at times because my inclination is always to put Josh's needs first, and I like to say we are both a work in progress.

Early

In the morning
before the light intervenes,

alters her posture

she knows she must soften today
with something more
than her usual passage,

a tending of her own heart
to calm her suspicion
that she has no choice.

Right now Josh is begging, "Please can we go to the church so I can hear the noon bells?" His decade-long fascination with the bells of St. Paul's Church in Augusta, Georgia, has taken OCD to a new level. I take him there once a week because I love him, and because it also serves as his reward for good behavior. And again, this church reminds me of that day, years ago, at Sweetwater, when nothing seemed impossible.

How to Finger Paint

Five year old hands
open like butterflies
finger paint earth
grab leapin' lime
ping pong lizard
dig dirt
tunneled treasures
circle beetle
all buggy-eyed
capture worms
squiggly giggles
pull dandelions
tickle chin

butter yellow
tuck in pocket
touch tall grass
crisp fall leaves
hands like petals
purple tulips
pink petunias
white gardenias
reach out
caress rain
slender spruce
slippery frogs
shiny stones
sunny terrain
reminds teacher

Maurine Meleck
(Friend of Team TMR)

18

YiaYia and Papou
Healing Harry

YiaYia

Chris and I are Harrison Conroy's grandparents and his mother's parents. We are very proud of our daughter Helen, who is a founding member of the Thinking Moms' Revolution, and our son-in-law Doug for the way they are tackling the symptoms of autism that came upon their son Harry starting at six months old.

We poured everything we knew into Helen when she was growing up and exposed her to everything we thought valuable in life. We taught her to be resourceful, pragmatic, and nonjudgmental until she gathered all the facts. When autism befell Harry, we saw her go into action to rescue him. There is nothing purer than the love of a mother for her child, and she showed not only that love, but also the courage and brilliance to persevere and educate herself to conquer the unknown. Chris and I have faith that Helen and Doug will find the answers to this problem and heal their child.

Chris and I decided that we would support Helen and Doug by listening to them and doing whatever they asked us to do for Harry. We never tried to run the show, but stood with them, and marveled, and gave thanks for the many and various treatments and therapies they tried. Each program worked to a point and brought Harry to a higher level; then they moved Harry on to the next step.

Harry was and is surrounded by love: from us, Doug's parents, his siblings, and his aunts and uncles. As a result of all this love, Harry loves us back. He has great eye contact and participates in all family events. We all applaud him and pay a lot of attention to him as he struggles to communicate. We know he is smart. We try not to frustrate him as we try to understand what he wants. I will say to you that he communicates with his eyes and we can almost read his thoughts. We do for Harry all the things grandparents do for their grandchildren. We don't differentiate between Harry and his brother and sister, though we do spend more time with him because we help Helen when the other children are in school, since Helen needs time to work on Thinking Moms' Revolution projects like this one. Fortunately, Harry's sister and brother are not jealous of him, because they seem to understand the situation. We don't interfere with G's or R's relationship with their brother. Harry can relate to each person by himself, and each relationship is different. I think this is very important and essential for a healthy family.

In seeing Harry learn to jump, climb, and ride a tricycle and then a two wheeler with training wheels, we learned tenacity and gained courage to push Harry to learn additional physical skills. At every turn, God placed the correct people in our path to help us, and we marveled at God's timing. Harry can swim and manage himself at our community pool. Often, as he jumps into six feet of water, I have to assure people not to worry or call 911, because Harry is a good swimmer. Helen is taking him ice skating, and he loves it. How strange this is—we live in southern Florida. Harry has a good command of his body and understands motor planning to acquire various skills. Presently, we are working on his fine motor coordination for writing and drawing. We are praying and waiting for Harry to talk consistently and in sentences, because he already knows many words. Even though I was an elementary school teacher for many years, working with Harry to help him learn to talk has given me a new appreciation of speech and language and all the skills involved in learning to talk (my grandson had seizures and apraxia and would gain and lose words regularly, which was so frustrating to him).

All this came later, however. Before the improvements, there were the symptoms and the diagnosis. When your adult child is faced with the evidence that his or her child, your grandchild, is on the autism spectrum, what can you do to be helpful to them? First, don't deny the findings. Accept that there is a problem and know that you don't have the solution in your back pocket. Humble yourself to your lack of knowledge on this topic and embrace your adult child, his or her spouse, and your grandchild with love and a positive attitude. Put away your pride and your ego and swing into survival and solution mode. Begin to read on the topic and learn as much as you can in a short time.

Encourage your adult child to read about the subject, research, and learn. Help them find the doctors and schools in your area that can help your grandchild. Find a support group in your area. There are many different methods of working with children with autism, and there are different strokes for different folks. Be patient until you find what works for your adult child's family and your grandchild. Remember this is their child, and you need to communicate gently and give them suggestions, not commands.

Even though you may have a vast store of wisdom, remember that you want to maintain a friendly relationship with your adult child and his or her entire family. It is better to really listen, ask questions, and comment later, after you think about what they have told you. Get involved in going to the therapy sessions and reinforce at home what your grandchild is learning at school. Babysit for the parents at least once a week so they can go out together and enrich their relationship. Become a real friend to your grandchild by getting to know him or her so that you can handle them when you are alone together. Know your strengths and limitations. Don't take on more that you can do. This is learned by trial and error.

If your physical strength is failing you, then work with your grandchild on other tasks, such as toys, painting, games, and puzzles. There is no one answer, but with prayer you will find your way to help. Don't let your feelings be hurt easily. Remember that your adult child is facing many problems and occasionally may take it out on you. Forgive and forget in the interest of positive results. Stay away from negative people and their opinions and don't argue with people or try to change their mind. This struggle is too personal to be discussed as a topic of interest.

Finally, pray, pray, and pray some more. The answers will come to you. Remember to laugh and enjoy your adult children and your grandchildren. Appreciate the good and the positive results and forgive the ignorant people you may encounter. Remember the angels that come your way to help you. Make sure you keep your friends and interests. Don't lose your personal life in this struggle, but be there. Most of all, be present.

Papou

Joan and I watched Harry and his twin sister when my daughter went back to work after their birth. I am a Greek grandfather, and I love to cook. It's how I show my love, so it was troubling that at only a few months old Harry began having feeding troubles. Everything from his bottle came back up. We introduced other foods a while later, but those came back up as well. The doctor told Helen he had reflux and put him on medicine for it, but it didn't really stop the problem. He would vomit and cry many hours of the day.

When Harry was eighteen months old, my wife and I took a long trip to Greece to bury my sister and attend a wedding. Helen called during the trip and informed us that Harry had been diagnosed with autism. Could that really be true? What did feeding problems have to do with autism? We returned not long after.

We all went on the Internet and scoured it for solutions. There were many suggestions for a gluten-free casein-free diet that seemed to be helpful for children with autism. I felt strongly about nutrition as Harry was so small and so sick and hated eating. I suppose if everything I ate burned my throat coming back up, I would hate eating too. Although Helen's doctor had said the GF/CF diet didn't work, we tried it.

Not even a full day after we removed dairy from his diet, Harry responded to his name for the first time in a year. We celebrated. Helen met with a nutritionist and swapped out milk for a mixture of coconut milk and a dairy-free product called "UltraCare for Kids," which, when combined, met the minimum standards for nutrition established by the USDA for infant formula. Harry's reflux disappeared, and we dropped the reflux medicine, but he still wouldn't eat.

Before we switched to the new diet, Harry often ate the following things: milk, yogurt, Cheerios, and gyro meat. Most things he ate, in fact, had dairy or gluten in them, and we believe they had contributed to his reflux. His throat must have burned so badly from those foods that he just hated trying to eat anything. Food was not pleasurable to him; he ate only when he absolutely had to. We had work to do.

Since I knew he loved gyro meat (which we learned sometimes had gluten in it), I started to develop a recipe that we could feed him to help him heal. I bought grass-fed, organic ground beef and started making a spaghetti sauce with it. I used only organic products, olive oil, herbs, and vegetables. We added rice. He ate it and could hold it down without vomiting.

After Helen had Harry tested and brought back lab results that showed some nutritional deficiencies (which go hand in hand with autism, as minerals are often not absorbed properly), I researched and slowly added foods into the mixture to give him the nutrients he needed. After about two weeks, he had regained strength and put on a tiny bit of weight.

Over time, as more test results came in, we adjusted for food sensitivities. Harry demanded sameness, so when we found out he was allergic to tomatoes, which he loved, we had to think about how we could make other food look the same. I substituted mashed sweet potatoes since they looked similar in color. The sweet potatoes were only a minor ingredient in his dishes, so the taste was acceptable.

This demand for sameness really compounded the feeding difficulties, since the texture, smell, taste, and even the way the food looked had to be the same, or he would not eat it. We walked a tightrope as we modified for low-manganese or low-piperine. The Great Asparagus Incident of 2012 will never be forgotten. Let's just say we got too daring adding veggies. He is not a fan of asparagus, and we had to eliminate all vegetables from his food for months to get him to trust us again and coax him back to eating. Months later, we slowly added them back in, starting with celery hearts, then expanding to include lots of white and light green vegetables that, when minced, didn't throw off the look of the food. Making these meals took a lot of time. I packed and froze two weeks' worth of meals at a time so that I was not cooking every day.

If you research foods and herbs, you will see that everything needed to heal is given to us by God. We just need to assemble the right combination for each child. I am happy to say that many of Harry's food sensitivities have decreased and that he has gained weight. His shoulders are now broad, and he has filled out. He may always be slim (after all, he does not like cookies or cake), but he is not sickly. His stomach is no longer bloated, he has not had reflux in years, and he is open to trying new things (sometimes).

I leave you my basic recipe below and ideas that we have used over the years. Read the labels on anything that comes out of a container.

Look into gluten-free, casein-free, and soy-free foods. Look at the Gut and Psychology Syndrome (GAPS) diet, which helps to heal the gut and which we needed to do for a while. Omit what doesn't work for your grandchild. We had to take out onions and garlic for a period of time because Harry tested sensitive to a substance in them. Food is a very important part of healing your grandchild, and if you like to cook, as I do, you too can help. Taking this on is such a key part of being involved, and it will be deeply, deeply appreciated by your child and, ultimately, your grandchild.

HARRY'S SPECIAL FOOD

Ingredients

2-3 tablespoons olive oil—preferably from Greece
1 large onion, finely chopped
4-5 cloves of garlic, finely chopped
5.5 lbs. 92% lean grass-fed sirloin
1 lb. zucchini, peeled, sliced lengthwise, and chopped to ¼ in. pieces
1 cup finely slivered and chopped to ½ in. celery hearts
Half of head of cauliflower, keeping soft stem on florets
2-3 sprigs of fresh oregano leaves, finely chopped
6-7 large basil leaves, finely chopped
2-3 sprigs of thyme, finely chopped
1 cup of fresh chopped parsley
Sea salt to taste
1 ½ cups rice or rice pasta, if tolerated

Add other vegetables as desired. We have used broccoli, carrots, and sweet potatoes, all with success.

Directions

Steam the cauliflower, zucchini, and broccoli, etc. until very soft.

Heat olive oil in a large pot. Add ground beef, onion, and garlic (if acceptable) and stir until it separates. Then add in celery. Add in the oregano, parsley, basil, and thyme and stir. Add in the vegetables and stir until they have a uniform texture. Add salt. Add five cups of water, stir, and cover. Stir frequently to avoid burning the bottom. When the water is mostly absorbed, set aside.

Cook rice or rice pasta (if tolerated) as directed and combine with the meat and vegetable mixture. Add or subtract as needed.

(When Harry's cholesterol was low, we added bacon and eggs to this mixture, undetected. We have used pinto beans at times for extra protein, and at one time used a sweet potato base. If tomatoes are tolerated, by all means make a meat sauce as the base.)

Once it cools, bag and freeze. Serve warm.

YiaYia and Papou

This has been a long road and a difficult journey, but we feel privileged to walk this road with Harry. We have never known love like this. Love for Harry and from Harry, as well as God's love, which is a fathomless fountain in a dry and thirsty land. To those readers in the same situation: we encourage you to give a listen to an old and familiar song written by Richard Rodgers and Oscar Hammerstein, who wrote it for their musical *Carousel* in 1945. It was performed in the musical by the aptly named character—Nettie Fowler. The song will remind you to "Walk on, walk on, with hope in your heart / And you'll never walk alone."

Christos and Joan Koronides
(Parents of Team TMR's Goddess)

19

Peaches
Autism Highway

ON THE ROAD OF LIFE, AS A GRANDMOTHER OF IDENTICAL TWIN BOYS affected by autism, I have met some truly incredible folks. I am so thankful for those who have helped my family along this journey. There has never been a more true statement than "It takes a village to raise a child." When you throw in a dose of autism, times two, you find out very quickly who will help you and who your real friends are.

The twins were born prematurely at twenty-nine weeks of gestation. Their birth weights were 1 pound 13 ounces and 2 pounds 3 ounces. They spent three months in the NICU. We really thought that their toughest battles had been won. Then came the autism.

I was in a near-fatal accident in August 2005, just six months before my grandsons were diagnosed with severe autism. While I was still recovering from my accident, their mom (my daughter) heard the words no parent should ever have to hear: "Your boys have autism." She tried to hold her grief inside to protect me. I tried to hold my grief inside to protect her. We struggled somehow through the next few years. Slowly, after lots of research, we have begun the healing process for these precious babies.

The grief still lingers today. The boys are now eleven years old. Yes, they still have autism. Family vacations have been replaced with treatments not covered by insurance to help them lead as an independent a life as possible. The words "save your money and start researching placement into a special home" have been replaced with hope.

I am not your typical grandmother. I am not called any cute grandmotherly names. I am simply "Ninny" to the twins. My daughter and the boys live with me. My home is not full of little knickknacks. Instead, it is filled with biomedical supplements and medicines, therapy toys, therapists, and more love than anyone could imagine.

My retirement days are not spent on a golf course or playing bridge at the senior center. They are spent advocating for families affected by autism. I may be working with our local sheriff's department, meeting with our governor or other state and federal lawmakers, or working with our school system. You will find me working to educate our politicians and advocating for effective autism insurance reform, as well as housing opportunities, job training, and employment opportunities for those affected by autism. In the last few months, I even branched out and started Tweeting. Yes, granny Tweets! Tweeting away so that those responsible for the autism epidemic will be held responsible and so that these two little boys will have a voice. Most nights, I get to cuddle with two lovable little boys. Those nights when I am so exhausted and frustrated, all I have to do is look into those beautiful eyes and somehow my strength is renewed to fight another day.

As I was writing this chapter, our home was less than a week away from foreclosure. Most folks never knew. Of course, because of that dreaded small-town local newspaper, the news did spread. One by one, all those wonderful people that we met on the autism journey stepped up to help us financially. With a lot of help from friends, our home did not go into foreclosure. It literally came down to just days. The funny thing is, today I feel rich! Not rich as in money in the bank or a stock portfolio, but rich as in surrounded by true friends.

No matter how good things are in your life, there is always something bad that needs to be worked on, and no matter how bad things are in your life, there is always something good you can be thankful for! You can focus on your purpose, or you can focus on your problems. If you focus on your problems, it is your problem, your issue, your pain. But one of the easiest ways to get rid of the pain is to get your focus off yourself and onto others.

I still have my moments of sadness, but I have learned to be thankful. Sometimes I still cry out, "Why?" and "Why the twins?" It took time for me to learn that the dark times are important to our faith. My experience has shown me that the thorns make the roses more precious. I do not resent the thorns. My battles pale compared to what the twins battle every second of the day. I look at my other grandchildren and feel so blessed. Hey, only two out of five are affected by autism!

I started working within the special needs community back in the mid-1970s. At that time, I worked with *one* family that had a child affected by autism. I remember very vividly that child's loud humming. I cannot recall his name, but that hum stayed with me all these years. In 2005, when not one, but both of my identical twin grandsons started the loud humming, I knew. What I did not put together at that time was that the humming was related to the toe walking, head banging, not sleeping, and constant diarrhea that followed their eighteen-month round of vaccines.

It was months before we could get a diagnosis for my grandsons. Even then, I refused to say the word "autism," as though everything would be all right if I just didn't say the word. Instead, our family heard that the boys would never talk, would never be potty trained, and that we should invest in placement into an institution instead of expensive therapies. It was a long ride home that day. Our beautiful blond-haired blue-eyed babies would have no future? NO WAY!!!

Before the term "Warrior Mom" became a buzzword in the autism community, this grandmother began researching. As I mentioned, I had been in a near-fatal accident just months earlier. I was not physically able to help care for my grandsons, but I could research. I became their warrior, determined that my grandsons would have a future and remain with the family that loves them.

I guess someone forgot to tell autism that I come from a long line of strong women. The farm that our little family lives on has been in my family for five generations. My grandmother became a widow at twenty-seven. She raised two little girls on these 400 acres with only a mule and sheer grit!

We started treating the twins with conventional therapies, such as speech and occupational therapy, the next week. Improvements soon followed. Then I came across Defeat Autism Now! on the Internet. My daughter thought the pain meds had done a number on me, until the twins' occupational therapist mentioned changing their diet to help ease their pain. What? My babies are in pain?

So we eliminated all corn and corn byproducts. No change. Then I was introduced to another new term, "GMOs" (genetically modified organisms). Next, we tried the gluten-free/casein-free diet, and we saw improvement. The twins still did not regain the words they had prior to that eighteen-month well-child checkup, but some of the crying stopped, and they started to sleep more.

Next, I had to find a doctor to help guide our next steps. At this point, my daughter was not totally sure whether I finally lost my mind or whether finding help was a reality. We finally found a Defeat Autism Now! doctor. The tests were done, and the reports opened everyone's eyes! They indicated high levels of aluminum and so many other chemicals that did not belong in our babies. Now grandma did not look or sound so crazy!

The evidence was finally accepted by the other family members—you know, the other grandparents and siblings that had thought I had flashed back to my hippie days. Family members shared videos of the twins before they were injured. Their uncle, an attorney, asked about filing a lawsuit. We had proof, right? Oh no! The manufacturers are protected! Wait, no one protected out babies? Anger!

After learning about the vaccine connection to autism, I couldn't help but wonder if my estranged ex-husband's military career played a role in my grandsons' autism. Because of his career, our children had to be vaccinated against yellow fever, cholera, and other diseases. I respect his service to our country, but there has to be a reason why the autism rate in military families is twice that of civilian families.

I roared to anyone who would listen. I lost friends along the way and made new ones. It seems like I went from a dirt road to a mega expressway. We began biomedical treatment, at great financial cost. But hope was finally starting to grow. Next, we focused on behaviors. We lost therapists along the way. The most trusted therapist that directed us to the DAN! approach informed us she could no longer work with the twins until their behaviors were addressed.

Off I went again to the Internet. I found new therapists, but all were expensive and none provided services in my rural area. After searching for what seemed like an eternity, we finally found one that proved helpful. It took seven years and several hundred thousand dollars, but we can finally go out in public. School is going better. Have the boys recovered? No, but we continue to have faith and hope. I'm now starting to think about a real future for the twins.

My daughter and I do not always see eye to eye, but I trust her motherly instincts. After experiencing the guilt, fear, and shame that followed the twins' diagnosis, she knows that autism does not change a mother's love.

And it has truly taken an entire village to help my grandsons. So many family members have contributed financially. They have listened when no one else would. In return, I have educated them—possibly ad nauseam—about autism: the characteristics, the signs and symptoms, the interventions, and the truly complex nature of the autism spectrum. But more importantly, I found I was educating myself in the process. It seems that I have spent every spare moment since the diagnosis immersed in a book about autism or collecting information online. My mission for truth has been renewed following the CDC whistleblower information that was made public in August 2014. I am dedicated to relentlessly seeking the truth! I still read medical literature and search the Internet. I study the autism success stories and the not-so-successful stories. I now realize that recovery looks different for each child, as do the effects and symptoms of the disease.

All the progress the twins have made would never have been possible if it weren't for the special people in my life and the doctors, therapists, teachers, and other acquaintances I have met on this journey. I've learned so much from TMR.

My retirement looks a lot different from how I had envisioned it. I am not traveling the world. Instead, I travel along that expressway called autism. Autism that came into our lives by injection, autism that we have been fighting, autism where hope is alive. Aidan and Gabriel are the bravest little souls I know, and they are living proof that recovery is possible. Maybe we haven't gotten there yet, but we are on the right expressway.

We all play many roles in our lives. My roles as mom to three children, grandmother to five, daughter, and friend, have been forever altered because of this journey. The way I view life has been changed forever. And yet, I've grown in a way I never imagined, and I have become stronger and more knowledgeable about autism than I ever thought possible.

This journey has been bittersweet. The journey that once seemed insurmountable and was often heartrending, filled with daily struggles and fear of the unknown, has turned into a recapturing of the moments I envisioned sharing with my grandsons.

To others dealing with similar struggles, I wish a journey filled with strength, love, and support from friends and families. We can do amazing things when we are put to the test! Most importantly, our grandchildren with autism are true heroes, and they do not need a cape to prove it. For all the medical testing they go through, for all the doctors' appointments and therapies they endure, for all the medications and vitamin concoctions we hide in their sippy cups, for all the squeezing to calm them down, for all the swinging to rev them up, they are really the true heroes in this war.

It is not easy on the heart or the wallet to be a "special" grandparent. I never knew, when the big "A" knocked on our door, what a turn my life was about to take. I will continue to research and learn. I will continue to educate others. But most of all, I will be the best supportive grandmother I can be. That is my mission now.

Sandi Marcus
(Friend of Team TMR)

Afterword
Jackie Goes Off

JACKIE GOES (MOTHER-IN-LAW OF LISA JOYCE GOES, THE REV) ADDRESSED a group of autism parents at the Give Autism a Chance Summit, 2014. Many of us were moved to tears by her words, and it was then that the Thinking Moms knew that a grandparents' book needed to be written. Jackie was introduced by Polly Tommey, Director of the Autism Media Channel, and founder of the Autism Trust USA and UK, and had this to say:

"Well, number one, you are amazing! Don't give up! Don't give up! You stay the course. You be strong like Galileo, and all those who have come before you, do not give up! As a grandparent, if I were talking to grandparents in this room, I'd say, number one, it's not about you, so shut up! [Applause.] Number two, we also need to grieve. You grieve twice. You grieve for your son, whom you dearly love. You grieve for his son. You watch him and his wife grieve. You take on a lot of their grief, and you pray. I happen to be a woman of faith, and I'm happy to say that Jesus Christ is my Lord and Savior, and that I trust him with their lives. I trusted this young man [her son Dave, the Rev's husband] when he was a baby into the Lord's arms. I trusted when he married his beautiful wife,

Lisa. We trust, and we move forward. You don't have time to cry, you get on with it.

"The other thing, as a grandparent . . . and hopefully if there is any grandparent out there looking or even caring . . . make your home a safe haven. Get rid of your shit, you don't need it. You make your home a safe haven. How many of you have ever been invited to someone's home for dinner with your autistic child? Probably not many; they don't know what to do with you. As a grandparent, you make it safe. You start getting into all this food stuff. You start to listen. You break down anything that's about you. You know, my dear people, I am on my way home, and I know it's not about me. I know it's not about my shit or my stuff. Let it go. So I pray that each one of you have old people who invite you in and let it happen. I have a piano that my dear son and daughter-in-law bought me. It was one of the three things I wanted in my life: a piano, a convertible (which they did not give me, but I did see someone drive up with one), and the third thing was an in-ground pool. But they gave me a piano, and that piano has more smudges on it, more crap on it, and is such a beautiful thing, because Noah, their beautiful son, my grandson, and I, we get to play it together.

"So I pray for all of you young people. I can't imagine the burden you have. But as a grandparent who dearly loves her grandson and my five others, and my husband who dearly loves all of us as well, we are supportive, we encourage. I have plenty of old people, friends, and I speak up. Old nurses, old docs, old colleagues—I was a teacher for thirty years. I speak up! Really, what do I have to lose? David said so eloquently one time, 'Sincerely, what do we have to lose?' You lose friends; hopefully you haven't lost your family.

"The other thing I am very proud of is this young man [her son, Dave]. I keep saying young, because to me he is, you all are; you're beautiful people. He has three other siblings, and that is so crucial. They're always talking about Noah. Always willing to do whatever it takes. And then there are the grandchildren that are not involved in their family, the grandchildren from another family. Inform them! This is what Noah is going to do when you come into his presence. So there is no fear.

"We love, and we love, and we love. That is why we are here. I used to teach theology to high school students, and one of the things I had on my bulletin board was 'The purpose to our lives is to learn to love, whatever that takes.' And you are called to learn to love in a different way. And I think it's just beautiful. As one of you said, 'If people are not on board, kick the dust from your sandals and move on.' Because there are many who need to hear, many who need to love, many in stores and so forth who need to understand what it is about and how it can be cured. Anyone who has ever had cancer does not sit around and say, 'Oh, isn't that just amazing, let's accept it.' Our grandchild was lost; there was no Amber Alert, there was no FBI, and we're mad as hell! Because we are going to find him, and so are you!" [Standing ovation.]